HOMEOPATHY

A Practical Guide to Everyday Health Care

Robin Hayfield

A GAIA ORIGINAL

Editor	Steve Parker
Design	Ellen Moorcraft
Illustration	Sally Launder Wayne Ford/Wild Life Art Agency
Picture Research	Kate Duffy
Managing Editor	Pip Morgan
Direction	Joss Pearson Patrick Nugent

First published in Great Britain in 1995 by
Virgin Books an imprint of Virgin Publishing Ltd
332 Ladbroke Grove, London W10 5AH

Printed and bound by Nuovo Istituto Italiano d'Arti Grafiche, Italy

A catalogue record for this book is available from the British Library.

ISBN 0-86369-818-2

10 9 8 7 6 5 4 3 2 1

HOW TO USE THIS BOOK

Homeopathy: A Practical Guide to Everyday Health Care can be used in several ways, according to your needs, and the way in which you approach health and illness. A full list of *Contents* is on the next two pages. There is also a complete *Index* on pages 141-143.

The *Introduction* describes the basis of homeopathy as a system of healing, and how it has developed into its modern form. General information on using homeopathy at home, pills, and prescribing is on pages 16-17.

Chapter One *Health and Well Being* covers important aspects of health care in our modern world, including diet, lifestyle, medical drugs, stress, and the importance of the immune system.

Chapter Two *Prescribing for Children: The Constitutional Types* gives information on a special type of homeopathic prescribing which you can carry out at home, and which is particularly suitable for children. It relies more on the personality and constitution of the individual child, than on the identity of the illness and its symptoms.

Chapter Three *Treating Common Ailments* is a practical guide to identifying and treating more than 50 common conditions and illnesses, ranging from high fever to deep depression. Pages 48-51 give general information on how to locate the ailment in the book and select a homeopathic remedy. There is a full list of ailments on page 53.

Chapter Four *A Guide to Remedies* provides profiles of about 60 commonly used homeopathic remedies, including all of those mentioned in Chapter Three. There is a full list of remedies on page 99.

The Home Homeopathy Kit on pages 138-139 describes a basic selection of remedies and other items for use at home, and how to store and use them.

Resources gives further information about obtaining remedies, and on suitable books, magazines, and training courses about homeopathy.

Contents

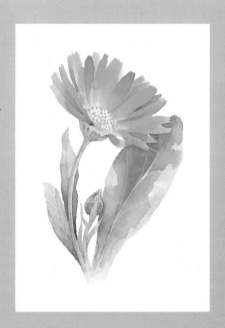

Introduction
What Is Homeopathy?   8

Chapter One
Health and Well Being   18

Chapter Two
Prescribing for Children:
The Constitutional Types   32

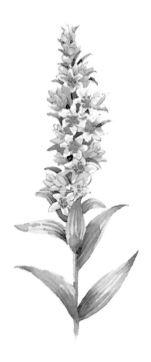

Chapter Three

Treating Common Ailments   48
    The Common Ailments   53
    Colds, Infections, and Fevers   54
    Digestive Problems   60
    Women's Problems   65
    Children's Problems   69
    Allergies   79
    Emotional Strains and Stress   82
    Accidents, Emergencies, and Injuries   85

Chapter Four

A Guide to Remedies   96
    Index of Remedies   99

The Home Homeopathy Kit   138
Resources   140
Index   141

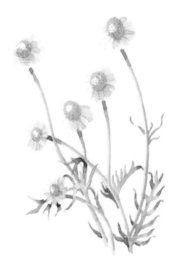

What Is Homeopathy?

Homeopathy is a system of medicine, that aims to relieve suffering, heal, and cure. It is safe and gentle, practical and easy to administer. It works effectively and equally well for males and females, for adults, children, and babies (and even animals). Homeopathy is also powerful. It can act very deeply on the body, over both the short and long term.

Homeopathy is based on a very simple natural principle. This is: "Like cures like." It means that any substance which has the power to harm the body, also has the power to cure – provided it is taken in extremely small, and therefore safe, doses.

"Similia similibus curantur –
Like should be cured by like."

German physician and chemist Samuel Hahnemann (1755-1843), the founder of modern homeopathy. This saying is a succinct summary of his system of medicine's central principle.

The importance of the symptom pattern

The principle of "like cures like" is best illustrated by an example. The homeopathic remedy Belladonna (see page 104) is prepared from a plant in the potato family found throughout Europe, called deadly nightshade. This is a tall, bushy herb with dark green leaves and long, purple, bell-shaped flowers. It favours chalky soils and grows well in hedgerows, woodlands, and thickets.

Deadly nightshade has large, glossy, seductive-looking black berries. Country people warn their children never to touch them. For the whole deadly nightshade plant is poisonous, and the berries are especially so. If a person eats just one or two berries, he or she would suddenly develop a characteristic and dramatic symptom pattern. Most of these symptoms are centred around the head. They may include a painful throbbing headache, which is made worse by bright light; a high fever,

The herb comfrey is the source of the homeopathic remedy Symphytum. As its country name of knitbone implies, it is used to help heal broken bones.

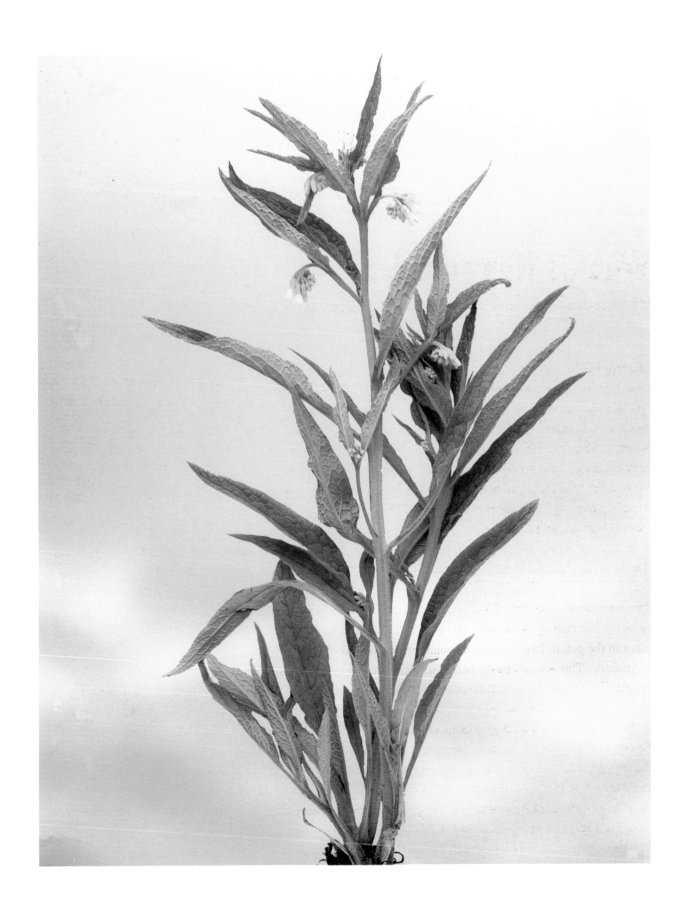

perhaps leading to delirium; a bright red face; palpitations and an accelerated heartbeat; skin that feels dry and burning; and very dilated or widened eye pupils. Despite the high temperature, there would be surprisingly little thirst.

The name deadly nightshade is very apt. The berries are as black as night, and a child may die after eating only three or four of them.

A force for good

Obviously, with such power to cause harm, deadly nightshade was a plant best avoided. But the homeopathic law says that "like cures like". So somewhere within the deadly nightshade is a force for good. Italian ladies of high fashion thought so. During the Renaissance period, they put tiny amounts of the berry juice into their eyes, to make the pupils dilate. This wide-eyed look made them appear more attractive and alluring, hence the name Belladonna or "beautiful lady". (Deadly nightshade's official scientific name is *Atropa belladonna*.)

The true healing power hidden within the plant is much more interesting and exciting. Once a substance has been "tamed" homeopathically, it can be used to heal the very symptoms which large doses produce in a healthy person.

Therefore, if you find you are developing a rapid and intense fever, and your face is red and dry, and feels burning, and your head throbs with pain – then take homeopathic Belladonna. Your symptom picture fits the one caused by deadly nightshade poisoning. Whatever the name of the disease that is causing the symptoms, Belladonna – in extreme and safe homeopathic dilutions – should help to relieve the symptoms, and restore you to health.

The history of homeopathy

The underlying idea of homeopathy has been known for at least 2,500 years. Around that time, its principles were mentioned by the Greek physician Hippocrates, the "Father of Medicine".

However, homeopathy has only been in use as a practical method of healing for about the last 200 years. The German physician and chemist, Samuel Hahnemann (1755-1843), rediscovered the principles

"Similar suffering" and the Law of Similars

The principles of homeopathy were known to the ancient Greeks. In fact the word *homeopathy* (sometimes spelled *homoeopathy*) was coined from two ancient Greek terms. These are *homoeo-* or *omio-* meaning "the same or similar", and *pathos* which means "hardship or suffering".

Homeopathy therefore means "similar suffering". This is another way of saying that "like cures like". Homeopaths call this underlying principle the Law of Similars.

and laws of homeopathy. He clarified and formulated them, and developed them into a practice of homeopathy which is very similar to the one we have today. He is rightly regarded as the founder of modern homeopathy.

Hahnemann set down the basic philosophy for homeopathy in a book called *The Organon*. It was first published in 1810, and Hahnemann revised it through six editions before his death. *The Organon* is still the bible of modern homeopaths. During his long life, Hahnemann introduced about 100 remedies, most of which are the core medicines still used today.

Since Hahnemann's time, homeopathy has certainly developed, and it has also waxed and waned in popularity. But the whole philosophy and practice of modern homeopathy springs entirely from the genius of his thoughts and experiments.

Hahnemann's insight

Hahnemann was originally trained as a doctor. But he soon became disillusioned, and even appalled, by the crude, unscientific, painful, and downright dangerous medical practices of the time. Much of this centred around blood letting, sometimes in excessive and fatal quantities, and the use of large doses of poisonous drugs, such as mercury. It is no exaggeration to say that the disease was often preferable to the cure.

Eventually Hahnemann gave up medicine for a time. To support his large family, he earned a small income from writing and translating – he was an impressive linguist, fluent in at least five languages. He also spent time trying to find a gentler, more effective way of healing, which would include a revival of the ancient beliefs in the benefits of good hygiene and fresh air.

His own "guinea pig"

In 1791, Hahnemann was translating an English article on the use of Peruvian or cinchona bark, also known as quinine. Quinine is a drug that is used in the treatment of the infectious tropical disease, malaria. Hahnemann became interested in this idea, and he started to experiment on himself. He consumed small pieces of the bark. Very quickly he developed a number of symptoms, including heart palpitations, drowsiness, alternating fever and chills, and drenching sweats. Each attack of symptoms lasted two or three hours, and reappeared at regular intervals.

Hahnemann had produced in himself all the symptoms of malaria, but without actually experiencing the disease itself. As soon as he stopped taking the bark, the symptoms disappeared. He had discovered a remedy, which we now call China (see page 110), and had rediscovered the Law of Similars (see page 11). From this, he reasoned that something in the bark could produce a symptom pattern that mimicked malaria – and the same mysterious something could treat the actual disease of malaria.

Testing the substances – the "provings"

Hahnemann now set about testing all sorts of substances, which he thought might contain curative powers. He experimented on himself and on his friends and colleagues, methodically recording the results for over 100 substances, which were then used to make remedies. This process of testing a substance on a healthy person to bring out the symptoms is called a "proving".

Since Hahnemann's original 100 provings, at least 2,000 more have been scientifically carried out. But in practice, only a few hundred remedies are regularly used by homeopaths.

Summaries of the symptoms produced by these substances have been listed, collected, compiled, and set out in books known as Materia Medica. There have been various versions of Materia Medicas prepared by a number of authors through the years. A Materia Medica and a Repertory – which is really a detailed index to the Materia Medica – are the two essential books that a practising homeopath always has by his or her side.

Shaking and dilution, again and again

Although Hahnemann had rediscovered the basic law of homeopathy, that "like cures like", there was still a problem. Many of the substances

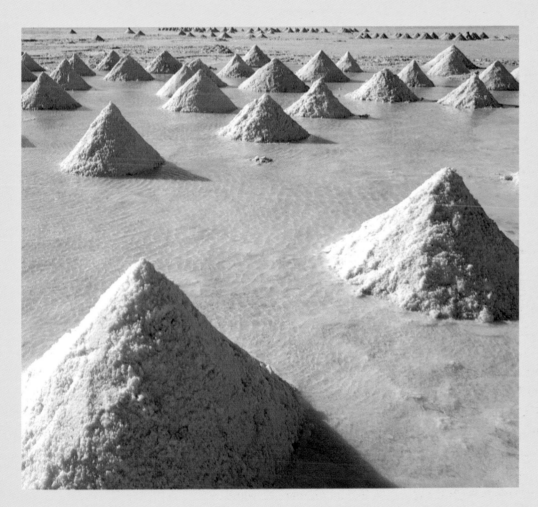

Salt is the raw material that provides us with the remedy Natrum muriaticum (Nat mur), one of the major remedies for grief and emotional traumas.

he wanted to use as remedies were very poisonous. Even in minute doses, there could still be risks and dangers. To avoid this, Hahnemann started to dilute the substances many times. Being a well-trained scientist, and an expert in pharmacy, he took great care in keeping the remedies pure and uncontaminated, as he made them into greater and greater dilutions. In fact, he diluted the remedies so many times that it seemed they could not possibly work. The dilutions were so weak that virtually nothing of the original substance remained!

Between each dilution, Hahnemann devised a method of vigorous shaking of the solution. This had a powerful effect and "energized" the remedy, releasing huge reserves of curative energy from the original mother substance. The vigorous shaking process is known as succussion. The combination of alternate dilution and succussion, at each stage of the remedy preparation, is called potentization.

The shorthand on the pill bottle

Homeopathic remedies are usually available as pills in bottles (see page 138). The bottle bears a label with the remedy name, and a number and a letter, for example, Arnica 6C. The number refers to the number of successive dilutions that have been carried out. The letter refers to the proportion or quantity of the dilution. For example, C stands for 100, which means that for each stage of the dilution and succussion process, one part of the previous dilution was added to 99 parts of water (or alcohol). Sometimes you see X, which means a dilution of one in 10, or M, which is 1,000C.

The combination of number and letter indicates the potency – the "power" or "intensity" of the preparation.

For Arnica 6C, one part of the original Arnica plant (see page 103) was first diluted in 100 parts of alcohol, and succussed. This process was repeated five more times. In the final dilution, there is only one part in 1,000,000,000,000 (one million million) of the original Arnica.

How does homeopathy work?

Once a remedy has been diluted beyond a potency of around 9C, the laws of chance and statistics say that not a molecule of the original

Scales of potency

In theory, the dilution-and-succussion process to produce homeopathic-strength remedies can be continued indefinitely.

In practice, there is a standard scale that runs 6C, 30C, 200C, 1M (1,000C), 10M, and even higher.

The 6C and 30C potencies are ideal for home use. The higher potencies are best left to qualified practitioners. This is because, as they become more dilute or weaker, paradoxically their effects become deeper and more powerful.

substance remains. The remedy includes nothing that could be called physical, so it cannot act directly on the physical body. Yet endless case histories show that homeopathic remedies do act effectively. So there must be something beyond the physical. We must be entering the realms of pure energy. The remedy seems to contain a "memory" of the original substance, in energy form. This acts on a non-physical "mysterious something" in the body.

The vital force

Hahnemann called this "mysterious something" the *vital force*. It is the spirit or "invisible driver" that, amongst other things, controls and regulates the body's self-healing mechanisms (see page 18).

The vital force is highly efficient and intelligent, and tries to keep the body as healthy as possible. Even illness happens for a very good reason. For example, a common cold is the body's way of clearing out toxins (poisons) and rebalancing itself. A fever is a sign that the body is fighting infection and burning up impurities, in much the same way as a good compost heap produces warmth and turns decay into renewal.

Skin diseases can be viewed as the body's way of keeping problems as far away as possible from the vital internal organs. Heavy, drug-containing creams can suppress this natural process and drive problems from the surface back into the inner body.

Acute and chronic illness

Usually the vital force copes very well with any problems. If it can, it throws them out as acute (short-term) ailments. If not, it may have to contain them as mild, chronic (long-term) illnesses.

Sometimes, however, the vital force – and therefore your body – becomes stuck. You may catch cold after cold, or develop chronic asthma, or suffer from persistent ulcers, or even cancer or heart disease. The vital force does what it can, and carries out a damage limitation exercise. But the situation may throw up an acute crisis, or a chronic and seemingly intractable problem.

At this point, outside help is required. This is where homeopathy can come to the rescue.

What symptoms tell us

Symptoms should not be regarded as the enemy, to be vanquished or suppressed at all costs. Orthodox medicine may approach symptoms in this way, but it does not tackle the root problem.

In homeopathy, symptoms indicate how the body is dealing with the problem. They also give vital clues to the type of outside help needed, such as rest, dietary changes, and which homeopathic remedy is needed.

A good homeopath is therefore like a good detective. He or she watches and observes, and tries to translate the symptoms into a picture of the required remedy. The homeopath notes the symptoms of the disease itself, and also the special way in which each individual person expresses those symptoms. In addition, the nature and the personality of the individual is taken into account. This complete picture is called the totality of symptoms, and it is part of the holistic view which is so important in homeopathy.

The individual picture

We are ill in different ways, even if the name of the disease is the same. Some people feel better in the cool, fresh air, while other prefer a warm, muggy room, even if they have the same illness. Certain children seem to be helped by cuddles and close contact, while others are so bad-tempered that you cannot get near to them!

These are different expressions of the vital force's distress. Each totality of symptoms points to the need for a certain remedy. In this way, homeopathy takes into account our individuality, which makes it holistic. An ailment can respond to one of many remedies, depending on the person's particular overall symptoms. Likewise, one remedy can cure many ailments, if the symptom picture fits.

How to use homeopathy at home

For chronic diseases and serious problems, consult a practitioner. However you can treat minor ailments and first-aid situations at home.
● *Minor injuries* Many small wounds and other injuries are easy to deal with. Use Arnica cream for bruises, or Calendula ointment for cuts

---

Homeopathy's "jump-start"

When you have a recurrent or persistent illness, it is rather like having a car with a flat battery. The car will not start under its own power. The only way to get the engine running again is a jump-start from another charged battery.

You can view homeopathy as giving a "jump-start" to the vital force of the body. With the correct remedy – the similar, as homeopaths call it – the body's own vital force and its self-healing processes can be given a boost from the outside. Soon you recover and regain normal health.

and sores (see pages 87 and 88). Minor first aid is usually straightforward, and the results are often surprisingly quick.

● *Considering the individual* The treatment of some ailments may need more thought. You will have to consider the particular characteristics of the problem for the individual person concerned. Some adults, and children in particular, show clear-cut personality traits and profiles, called constitutions. These are are amenable to the process called constitutional prescribing (see page 32).

● *Ailments and remedies* Locate the problem at hand in the chapter on common ailments (see page 53). Here the ailments are described, and likely remedies indicated. When you think you have found the correct remedy, you can double-check its symptom picture in the remedy section (see page 99).

● *Wrong remedies* Do not worry if you think that you have used the wrong remedy. Homeopathy is very safe and the pills have no side-effects, which is worth remembering if a child gets hold of a bottle. If a remedy does not work, try the next most likely remedy on the list.

● *Changing remedies* In an emergency, you can repeat the remedy every 15 minutes. Or you can change to another one if the first one does not work. Otherwise, it is wise to wait a few hours or overnight, before you change remedies.

● *Maintaining remedies* If you find a remedy that works well, and the symptom picture does not change, then stick with that remedy. Repeat it if necessary (for doses, see pages 48-51).

● *The gentle approach* Use homeopathy lightly. You are trying to help your body heal itself. Once your body seems to be coping well, and you are feeling better in yourself, then you only need to watch and wait. Only if a sense of "stuckness" reappears, do you need to intervene with another remedy. If in doubt, trust your vital force or seek advice.

● *Unsuitable ailments* Homeopathy can be used for most ailments which produce symptoms. The main exceptions are mechanical problems such as dislocations, back problems, and severe physical injury, and certain other intractable conditions.

● *Advantages* Homeopathy is safe, gentle, and convenient, with no side-effects. Children and animals respond particularly well. The remedies are easy to obtain (see pages 139-140).

Homeopathy is an art as well as a science. It is fascinating, rewarding to use, and becoming increasingly popular all over the world.

Chapter One

Health and Well Being

The human body is a beautifully designed, intricate system. It is governed by the most intelligent computer imaginable – the brain. This has been partly pre-programmed at birth, through the genes inherited from the parents. But it is also ready to learn immense amounts of information and adapt to endlessly different situations.

On occasions, the body becomes ill or develops other problems. When this happens, it has an internal self-adjusting process that comes into play, to heal itself. It usually succeeds. Only in rare cases does the self-healing mechanism seem to fail. This may be due to faulty genes, or a severe accident, or prolonged lack of care. When the body becomes weakened and "stuck" in this way, it may benefit from outside help.

Homeopathy is one of the helpers. It is a way of healing that respects the body as a delicate and complete system. Used carefully, homeopathy can provide help by loosening the sticking point, and allowing the body's own self-healing processes to work once more.

The importance of the individual

Every human being is an individual, with individual needs – a seemingly obvious fact. We all recognize the truth of this statement. Yet when we consider our physical and emotional well being, we seem to pay it scant attention. For example, we do not all need the same diet. We do not all sleep the same number of hours each night. We do not cope equally with life's stresses and strains. And when we fall ill, we do not all need identical medicines or treatment.

"In a state of health, the spirit-like vital force which animates the body, reigns in supreme sovereignty."

Samuel Hahnemann, founder of modern homeopathy, in his major work *The Organon* (first published in 1810).

Some homeopathic remedies have different effects on different individuals. However, Calendula, made from the marigold plant, has a universal application for healing open wounds.

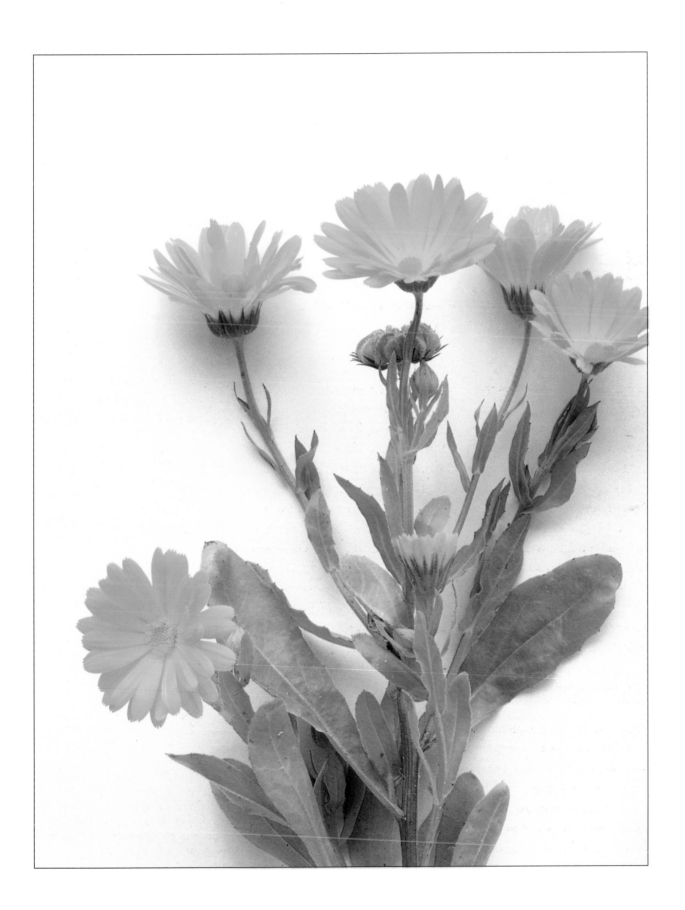

Susceptibility

Most people have their weaknesses or sensitive points. This feature is known as "susceptibility". The susceptibilities are part of each person's constitution – the individual's unique make-up of physical, mental, and emotional characteristics (see page 32).

A susceptibility may be emotional, as in a very sensitive person who has a nervous breakdown after losing a loved one. It may be physical, as in the vulnerable child who becomes handicapped after a routine vaccination. It may be functional, as when a person develops a dangerous allergic condition after eating a food which is happily tolerated by others, such as almonds, or the gluten in wheat.

Some children always seem to catch a chill after getting wet. Others develop colds that usually go down to their chests. Certain adults are susceptible to heart disease or cancer, while others remain well until arthritis catches up with them in their seventies.

You can try to recognize your susceptibilities by observing what your body is telling you. Then you can start to make the necessary changes in your life that help to turn your weaknesses into strengths. For instance, you can make changes for a healthier diet, and alterations to your lifestyle so that you do not become over-stressed.

You can use homeopathy by self-prescription for minor situations, as described in Chapter Three. In addition, you can also employ the skills and prescribing experience of a homeopathic practitioner, who may be able to boost your energy systems and lessen any susceptibilities.

Threats to the body and mind

We live on a very polluted planet. Our bodies are being continually bombarded with substances that we have not been programmed to cope with or accept. Our air and water are no longer pure. The earth is poisoned with pesticides and artificial fertilizers, heavy metals and radiation. Our food is adulterated with additives, and much of its goodness and vitality has been processed out.

We are given unnatural drugs such as antibiotics and steroids, which may steadily weaken our immune systems (see page 26). We suffer too much electromagnetic radiation from pylons and transformers outside

Looking after yourself

Some people are born with an "iron make-up". They may seem to survive well, even though they eat a poor diet, take too much alcohol, or do too little exercise. True, there is great individual variety in our basic make-up. However, people with apparently tough bodies may well pay the price in later life. There is often a long time period, perhaps many years, between abuse and illness, as in arteriosclerosis (hardening of the arteries) or cirrhosis of the liver. It is therefore wise to alter faulty lifestyle early, to avoid trouble later.

the home, and from television sets and computer screens inside. Many of us also damage ourselves through smoking tobacco, misusing drugs, and drinking too much alcohol.

Our uncontrolled emotions and mental attitudes can also cause us physical illness. Few people can cope with extreme stress for long. It forces an unnatural rhythm on the body, which upsets the healing process. Persistent negative emotions such as greed, jealousy, excessive anger, guilt, and lack of self-worth can also play havoc with health.

Fortunately, if you recognize and consider these threats in time, you can choose to do something about them – and be well. With information in books such as this one, you can empower yourself, and take responsibility for your own health and well being.

How much stress?

Moderate levels of stress, now and again, are a natural fact of life. They should cause no harm to an otherwise healthy person. Stress is an essential part of your survival mechanism. It prepares your body for rapid action, and gets you ready to avoid or escape from dangerous situations at great speed.

But continual exposure to very stressful situations over a prolonged period can cause deep depression and anxiety. It may even lead to a complete breakdown in health. This can happen if you are in an unhappy and destructive relationship, or if you have a dictatorial parent, employer, or teacher, or if you are in any situation that breaks down your sense of self-worth and self-respect.

Severe, prolonged stress such as this should be dealt with, otherwise the resulting illness may prove difficult to cure. It is rather like trying to climb up a down-moving escalator. Homeopaths call this problem "a maintaining cause". You either have to adapt to the situation – or change it. Sometimes the appropriate homeopathic remedy can give you the energy boost, to help you make the change.

Action on stress

* Find a quiet place where you can be alone for five or ten minutes each day. Allow your mind to remain quiet at this time. Become aware

of your physical body and its sensations. Try to get in touch with the still, calm centre that lies deep within each of us.

* Let nature take some of the strain. Take up gardening, grow houseplants, or walk in the park or countryside. Flowers and trees have great natural powers to soothe a troubled human spirit. Indeed, many homeopathic remedies are prepared from them.

* Join a yoga, relaxation, meditation, or exercise class.

* Seek help from a kind and sympathetic friend.

* Consult a professional counsellor or a homeopath.

* Try some of the homeopathic remedies for stress (see page 82).

* Remember that prolonged, unrelieved suffering is not good for the soul. Somehow and somewhere, a change is always possible.

Medical drugs

Homeopaths believe that wherever possible, the body should be allowed to cure itself, through its own natural healing resources (see page 18). If this does not seem to be happening, then alterations in habits, lifestyle, diet, and other factors may be considered. In addition, homeopathy can be used to stimulate the natural healing mechanisms.

In general, we use far too many drugs. Some are not very efficient at what they are supposed to do. Others are inherently poisonous, with unpleasant or even dangerous side-effects. Many have unknown long-term effects. Certain drugs may weaken the immune system, so that the body's self-healing qualities become "lazy" (see page 26). Lowered powers of immunity can allow chronic illness to take hold, which leads to more drugs, and it becomes a vicious circle.

This is not to say that we should never take drugs. Antibiotics can save lives in desperate situations. With our present state of knowledge, there is no alternative to insulin for certain cases of diabetes. But no drug is totally safe. Even the humble aspirin can cause ulcers and dangerous stomach bleeding if taken over a prolonged period.

Action on drugs

* If you are advised to take a course of drugs, especially over a long period, make sure that you fully understand the whole process. Ask the

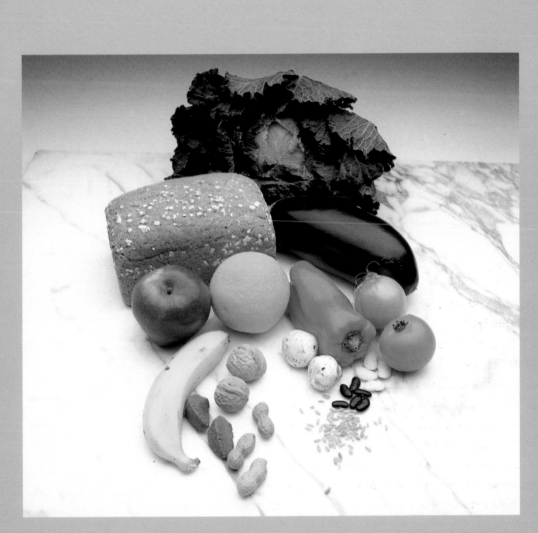

The elements of a good diet include fibre or roughage. Along with valuable nutrients, fibre is plentiful in unrefined wholemeal grains and their products, such as breads and pastas, and in fruits and vegetables. Fibre does not contribute any actual nutrient substances to the body. But its physical presence keeps the digestive system working smoothly and healthily.

doctor three important questions. What are the possible side-effects? What is the likely outcome, and is it worth any drawbacks? And – not *are* there any alternatives – but *what* are the alternatives? (You can use the same approach if you are being advised to have a surgical operation.)

* If you have worries or doubts, or if you suspect that you have not been given the full story, get a second or even a third opinion.

* Explore other possibilities, such as a change of diet, or massage, or exercises. Talk to a homeopath or other holistic practitioner. Enquire if there is a safer and gentler alternative. Very often, there is.

The importance of diet

"We are what we eat" – a saying that is so familiar, few of us appreciate the truth which lies behind it. Food provides the raw materials from which your body is made and maintained. And lest we forget, food also provides the raw materials from which our children's bodies will be made. Good, fresh, wholesome, nourishing, unprocessed, and generally natural foods produce healthy human beings.

The reverse is equally true. Too many processed, treated, preserved, and junk foods create junk bodies. Almost all modern diseases, including many cancers and certain types of heart problems, have been linked to bad eating habits.

Action on diet – the "don't"s

* Don't eat too many processed foods. This usually means you should avoid eating out of packets, cartons, and tins.

* Don't eat too much salt, or too much sugar.

* Don't eat too much refined carbohydrate, as in white rice, or refined flour, as in white bread. Choose the unrefined, wholefood versions.

* Don't eat too much animal fat, which is contained mainly in red meats, fatty types of meats, and certain dairy products.

* Don't drink too much tea or coffee.

* Don't eat foods that contain lots of additives. Read the packet to see which additives, preservatives, and other chemicals are present.

* And for the sake of your weight and waistline, don't overeat.

Essential nutrients

Certain essential nutrients are vital for good health. The main nutrients include minerals and trace elements, proteins, vitamins, carbohydrates (sugars and starches), fats (essential fatty acids), and fibre or roughage.

Eat a widely varied diet, and you should not be short of essential nutrients. However, in reality, there is a risk of certain deficiencies – especially vitamins and trace elements. If you suffer from a persistent or chronic problem, investigate your diet further, perhaps by consulting a nutritionist.

Action on diet – the "do"s

* Eat plenty of fresh fruit and vegetables. If you can eat organic produce, even better. Include the (washed) skins of fruit and vegetables, since many of the nutrients are stored there. Take plenty of fresh, leafy vegetables such as spinach and cabbages. Onions and garlic are also very good. Try and eat a raw salad every day.
* Cook your food lightly, and especially your vegetables, to avoid losing essential nutrients. Steaming or stir-frying is better than prolonged boiling or deep-frying.
* If you fry food, do so in unprocessed vegetable oils, such as olive, corn, or sunflower oil. Extra virgin olive oil is particularly suitable.
* Include plenty of wholegrains in your diet. These include wholemeal bread and brown rice, which will provide you with fibre as well as essential nutrients. Choose organic products if you can find them.
* Substitute fish or poultry for red meats, when you can.
* A wholefood vegetarian diet can be particularly healthy.

Changing patterns of disease

The nature of disease has changed dramatically over the past 150 years. The scourges of the last century were largely the acute (sudden-onset) infectious diseases, such as measles, tuberculosis (TB), cholera, typhoid, diphtheria, and scarlet fever. These diseases have been in steep decline for most of this century. They are now rare in most industrialized or Westernized countries.

The decline of these infectious illnesses predates mass immunization. Rather, it has been attributed to better living conditions, cleaner drinking water, more hygienic and efficient sewage systems, and a general improvement in diet and nutrition. In addition, the bacteria, viruses, and other microbes which cause these familiar diseases seem to have lost much of their virulence.

Today in the industrialized countries, we suffer from a different set of ailments. Allergy-based problems such as eczema, asthma, and hayfever – almost unknown in the 19th century – are now possibly the fastest-growing of all disease groups. Likewise, cancers and heart disease are very much 20th-century phenomena in Western countries.

Is this progress? It seems that we have swapped one set of problems for another. However, there has been a change in the basic pattern of illness. People formerly suffered a number of violent, acute, contagious diseases. These could be very dangerous in the short term – especially for children – although they were far from universally fatal. People today suffer a large number of chronic, long-term, persistent problems, which are largely incurable by modern orthodox medicine.

Disease and the immune system

One worrying aspect of this change in disease pattern involves the immune system – the body's self-healing mechanism. This is a body-wide network of microscopic cells, natural body chemicals, and channels for energy flow, which is stunning in its complexity and sophistication. It monitors the body for invasion by unfamiliar or foreign particles, mainly germs. Or it reacts against usually harmless substances such as pollen grains, to which the body has become hypersensitive, or allergic.

As soon as these foreign substances appear in the body, the immune system swings into action with a complex series of defence reactions, to destroy or disable the invaders. The battle produces the symptoms of the infection or allergy.

The patterns of modern diseases suggest that our immune systems are losing their former ability to shake off disease. We often manage only to contain, rather than defeat, the problem. Our general health and vitality may become lowered, by factors such as poor diet, too many drugs, prolonged stress, and lack of exercise, as described on the preceding pages. We feel fatigued and below par for much of the time.

The role of natural immunity

What does the decline in infectious diseases tell us about immunity? In the last century, a proportion of the population succumbed to the major infections. But many other people survived by developing natural immunity. Moreover, the natural or boosted immunity could be passed from mother to baby, by breastfeeding. So babies were especially protected in the risky early months.

Of course, none of us want a return to those dangerous times. But homeopaths tend to look at childhood infectious diseases – notably measles, mumps, and chickenpox – in a different way to the orthodox view. Most homeopaths contend that the infectious diseases are seldom dangerous to a healthy child, and that to catch them is quite natural. Through the process of developing and then conquering the infection, the child gets rid of inherited and acquired toxins (poisons) from the body, and also gets a generous boost to the immune system.

Problems for the immune system

With the appearance of AIDS in the 1980s, public consciousness has become much more aware of the role of the immune system. AIDS is Acquired Immune Deficiency Syndrome. It is not actually a disease in itself. No one dies directly from AIDS. However, as a person develops AIDS, his or her body's immune system becomes very weakened. It can no longer fight off infections, cancers, and other illnesses. The potential for self-healing is exhausted. Without its self-protecting mechanism, the body succumbs to these illnesses.

Usually, AIDS follows infection with HIV – the Human Immunodeficiency Virus. The condition of being infected with HIV is called "HIV positive". There is often a long period, ten years or more, between acquiring HIV, and the development of the illnesses which indicate so-called "full-blown" AIDS.

Yet some people have been HIV positive for much longer than the typical period, and remained healthy, without developing AIDS. It seems that by changing lifestyle and attitudes, AIDS can be kept at bay.

There are also a small number of people with full-blown AIDS who have managed to boost their immune systems to such an extent that they have survived for a relatively long time. Similarly, there are cases of people with serious, even terminal, cancer who have suddenly and dramatically shown an improvement, known as spontaneous remission.

The immune system under threat?

Perhaps the decline in childhood infectious diseases, and the corresponding rise in more chronic and persistent problems such as allergies, do not bode well for us and our children. Asthma (see page 70) is a particularly worrying example. Thirty years ago, most schools in a major city such as London seldom had an asthmatic child. Currently, in some urban areas, as many as one child in five is classed as asthmatic, and the proportion is still rising.

We may attribute problems such as allergies to trigger factors, such as milk or wheat in the diet, or pollen or airborne products of the house-dust mite. But these are merely the stimuli or triggers which bring on an attack. We have to look behind these triggers, or secondary factors, to find the real causes. In many cases, evidence points to a weakened or depressed immune system.

Why are our immune systems and self-healing processes in such a poor state? It is human nature to search for a scapegoat outside ourselves, rather than look inward. However, it seems likely that the answer lies in a combination of factors.

Pollution

It is fashionable to blame environmental pollution for almost anything, and there can be little doubt that this is an important ingredient in a cocktail of causes. Recent research suggests vehicle exhaust fumes, in particular, as a major contributor to allergic and immunity problems.

But pointing the finger at pollution is by no means the entire story. New Zealand, with some of the cleanest air in the world, also has one of the highest rates of asthma. Remember that atmospheric pollution has been around for a long time, although it has become less visible. Yet, as we swap smoking chimneys for vehicle exhausts, we have also exchanged bronchitis for chronic asthma. The pollution may well affect the body's powers of self-protection and self-healing.

Diet, drugs, and the immune system

The quality of our food (see page 24) is certainly another factor. It looks clean and germ-free, processed and preserved, and encased in its hygienic wrapper on the supermarket shelf. But it is far removed from its natural growing place and state. Its life and vitality have long since diminished. The removal of essential nutrients from food, through

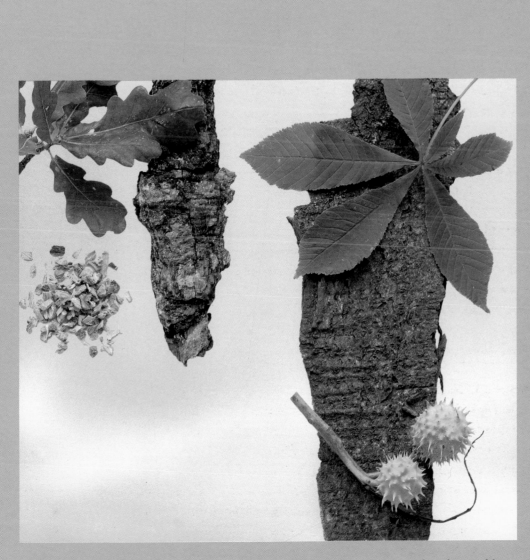

The large brown nuts or "conkers" of the horse chestnut tree, contained in the prickly green cases (right), yield the homeopathic remedy Aesculus. This is helpful, along with dietary changes, for curing digestive lower-bowel disorders such as haemorrhoids. The oak tree (left) also has curative properties.

processing, can lead to subtle dietary deficiencies – which again may help to depress the body's immune system.

Homeopaths and other natural healers also feel concerned about the excessive use of orthodox drugs by the medical profession (see page 22). We are filled with antibiotics, steroids, vaccines, tranquillizers, and many others, that are so often over-prescribed. Once again, such unnatural input into the body can weaken the immune system.

The 20th-century lifestyle

Another factor in the cocktail of causes is our lifestyle and values in the 20th century. Indigenous peoples who have not deserted their traditional ways of life, and who live simply in surroundings close to nature, do not suffer from the chronic diseases prevalent in the West. These people tend to live in stable, extended family groups, often with strong religious or spiritual ties.

In stressful situations, support is readily available from family and close friends, who are usually living nearby. In times of sorrow, they do not grieve alone.

When such people move into the Westernized attitudes and lifestyle, they seem to leave their natural immunity behind. They soon develop the diseases associated with Western civilization.

The importance of attitude and being cared for

In the quest to "conquer disease", our modern scientists study the diseases and the people who are sick with them – but not the people who are healthy, and who seem to stay healthy. Surely some of the answers lie with them?

People who are determined to get well and stay well, who feel cared for, and whose self-esteem is high, seem to stand a better chance of staying healthy. If illness strikes, they also have a higher likelihood of overcoming it more quickly and more completely, compared to people who lack this determination.

As further evidence, there are reports of orphaned children who are born HIV positive, having received the virus from their mothers during birth. Their immune systems are weakened. But if such a child is placed

Check list for a healthy life

* Eat a healthy, balanced diet.
* Get regular exercise and sleep.
* Avoid prolonged stress.
* Avoid toxic and unnatural substances, especially processed foods, excessive sugar, and tobacco.
* Use homeopathy or other natural healing, wherever possible.
* Take responsibility for your own health. It's your body. Gain the confidence to cope.
* If you need help from a health practitioner, find one that you trust, and who empowers you.

with loving, caring foster parents, then he or she has a greater chance of thriving and becoming healthier.

The vital force and healing energy

We understand very little of the human mind, and only the basic mechanics of the human body. This quest for complete understanding is a fine challenge, but perhaps it is ultimately fruitless. The body and mind continually renew themselves as they adapt to new situations. Even if we could understand more of the body's mechanics, we might never be able to locate its "invisible driver" – the vital force (see page 15), which controls and guides its natural healing and immune systems.

Modern physics tells us about the interchangeable nature of matter and energy. It is expressing, in a different way, what mystics through the ages have always told us. The physical body is an illusion. It is really a massive and complex web of subtle energy. To heal deeply and completely, therefore, it makes sense to use similar types of energy. Once again, homeopathy can help, because it is an energy medicine.

The sources of healing energy

In many cases of illness, you may find that the healing energy is produced by your body's own resources, and organized by its "invisible driver". It may also be possible to change your mental approach and attitudes, and perhaps re-programme your immune system, by sheer force of will.

In other cases, the extra energy to heal is sought outside the body, from homeopathy, herbs, massage, or similar therapies. The energy acquired can bring recovery and cure providing the basic cause is dealt with. In the long term, it can also help you to change your attitudes, values, and habits, to promote permanent healing.

But perhaps the greatest source of healing energy can be obtained in a simpler way. The evidence is shown by the indigenous person with a plot of land, and with family and friends nearby. It is also revealed by the AIDS orphans who are now cherished by their new parents. This source is simply loving care.

Chapter Two

Prescribing for Children: The Constitutional Types

If you consult a qualified homeopathic practitioner about a particular ailment or problem, you will probably find that she or he will begin by asking you all manner of varied questions. When you first hear these, you may think that the questions, and the answers you give, are completely unconnected with the problem at hand.

For example, you are likely to be asked about your food preferences and eating habits, your body temperature and how it varies, your worries and anxieties, your emotional nature – such as how you feel about love and anger – and so on.

But you should consider the questions seriously and answer them truthfully. The information is important and relevant. Homeopathy is far more than simply considering symptoms or problems in isolation, such as a headache, or a cough. The answers that you give to these wide-ranging questions will allow the trained homeopath to put together a clearer, more holistic profile of you as a person.

> "Unless causes are removed from beginning to end, the disease can reproduce itself ... The totality cannot be removed without removing the cause."
>
> Dr James Tyler Kent (1849-1916), the homeopath who developed the notion of constitutional prescribing.

Your constitution

This profile of you as a person, in turn, provides the homeopath with some knowledge of your whole constitution. The "constitution" is not limited to describing the physical body, and the strengths and weaknesses in its various systems. It also applies holistically to deeper parts of you, including problems that have weakened or otherwise affected your immune system (see page 26) and thereby possibly caused your illness. Your type of personality and your psychological processes

The lime in the common oyster's shell is the source of the remedy known as Calcarea carbonica, or Calc carb. This is one of the major constitutional remedies (see page 36).

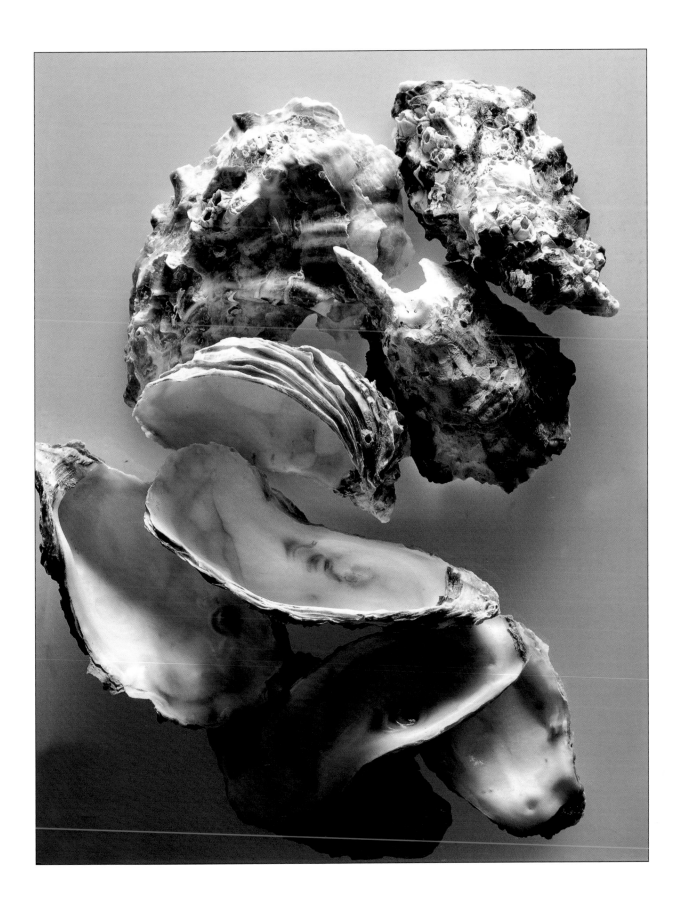

are also of the utmost importance. Thus your constitution is a complex combination of physical, mental, and emotional factors.

Constitutional remedies

Knowledge of an individual person's constitution can then lead to the identification of a remedy which acts very deeply on that individual's whole system. This is known as the constitutional remedy for that particular person. The remedy can help not only for the symptoms and ailments that it treats in general prescribing. It can also help with a wide range of other problems and ailments.

A drawback to this type of self-prescribing is that constitutional remedies are not always easy for the inexperienced to find or identify – especially for adults. Constitutional self-prescribing at home, without professional help, is generally difficult, because of the complexities of an individual's physical and mental make-up. Normally, the skills and experience of a homeopathic practitioner are required.

However, home constitutional prescribing for children can be more successful. This is because a child's personality tends to be less complex and developed, and more "transparent", compared to an adult.

Personality portraits

The following pages describe profiles or portraits for six basic types of constitution in children. There are many more, but the six given here are probably the most common, and the easiest to identify.

Mixtures of constitutional types occur. However, in many children, one type predominates.

Each personality type includes a list of key points as a "picture" for the remedy. If this remedy picture fits your child, then you can use that remedy for all sorts of ailments which your child may have, or even as a general tonic. You may find the constitutional remedy useful in chronic (long-term) states – for example, for the child who is prone to earaches, or who is always getting colds.

Constitutional prescribing for children requires that you think of your child in a different way. Your reserved, emotionally suppressed six-year-old child could be a Nat mur type, and may respond to that remedy for a wide variety of ailments. A clinging, whining baby could be a Pulsatilla type, and so be cured by Pulsatilla.

Dosage

When your child feels unwell, with any minor symptoms or illness, give one 30C pill of the constitutional remedy daily. Continue until he or she feels better, but do not use a remedy for more than one week.

Or you can give the constitutional remedy as a one-off 30C tablet, as a "pick me up" if the child seems tired, vague, or otherwise off colour.

SUMMARY OF CONSTITUTIONAL TYPES

Sometimes the constitutional types are unclear and blurred at the edges, and may even seem to overlap. This chart helps you to compare directly the six main types and decide, on balance, to which group your child belongs. You can always revise your judgement and try another, related constitutional remedy. Some children change their type as they grow and develop.

Key Calc carb features

- Methodical and deliberate, perhaps to the point of appearing slow and stubborn
- May be quite plump and sweaty
- A liking for starchy foods
- Independent, yet not very adventurous

Key Nat mur features

- Very sensitive to comments and criticisms, however well meaning
- Suppressed or locked-up emotions that only show in private
- Wise and serious beyond her or his years
- Self-contained and independent

Key Pulsatilla features

- Fear or worry of being abandoned
- Particularly sensitive to events such as changing school
- Indecisive and changeable, which includes moods, food preferences, and symptoms
- Delicate, shy appearance
- Prefers cool, fresh air

Key Lycopodium features

- Shy, lacks confidence, anxious, worried
- Fear of being seen to fail
- Craving for sweets and sugary foods
- Tendency to produce intestinal gases or wind

Key Phosphorus features

- Slightly delicate and fine looking
- Warm, affectionate personality
- Responds well to love and affection
- May lack concentration and be easily distracted
- Weak points include stomach, throat, and chest
- Often of a nervous disposition

Key Sulphur features

- Confident, active, outgoing
- Sometimes self-centred and insensitive to the needs of others
- Physically big, strong, and boisterous
- Untidy, scruffy, even messy, in both appearance and habits
- Does not feel the cold

IS YOUR CHILD A CALC CARB TYPE?

Personality

Calcarea carbonica (Calc carb) children like to do things at their own speed and in their own way – which is usually rather slowly and methodically. This is also the way and the pace at which they tend to learn.

As a consequence, they may become very unhappy if they are pressured or rushed, even to the point of throwing rages and temper tantrums.

Another effect of this personality is that the Calcarea carbonica child may appear to be obstinate and rigid. But really, she or he simply needs to understand the whys and wherefores, before taking any actions.

A third consequence is that because of the fairly slow and deliberate progress, Calcarea carbonica types may be late developers. But they are usually just as intelligent as other children, so by the end of the process, they achieve average or above-average results.

Typical Calcarea carbonica children are independent and quite serious. Yet they are usually contented, happily playing on their own when left to their own devices. Generally they are easy going, if not prodded too much.

> *Key Calc carb features*
>
> • Methodical and deliberate, perhaps to the point of appearing slow and stubborn
> • May be quite plump and sweaty
> • A liking for starchy foods
> • Independent, yet not very adventurous

Fears and worries

Calcarea carbonica children are not normally the adventurous types. They need to feel safe and secure. So they can easily become alarmed by the darkness, by monsters on television or in books, or even by mice or spiders.

Physical features

The Calcarea carbonica child is usually quite plump, and also rather sweaty – especially on the hands and head. The perspiration means that the pillow may become damp at night.

Likes and dislikes

These children love stodgy, starchy foods such as bread and pasta. They may also crave eggs, especially soft-boiled ones. Babies may want to eat chalk or earth.

Yet they often dislike meat, and milk and milk products tend to disagree with their digestion. They may be sensitive to the cold, and like to keep their heads warm, such as by wearing a hat.

Symptoms and illnesses

* Calcarea carbonica types are prone to constipation, although this does not seem cause them any great problems or upsets.

* The ankles may be a weak point, and prone to sprains and strains.

* There may be a tendency to colds, coughs, sore throats, and other minor respiratory ailments, often brought on by damp and cold conditions.

* They may get fevers with a high temperature. These fevers characteristically respond to Belladonna as an acute or fast-acting remedy.

* As a constitutional remedy, all sorts of problems can be helped by Calcarea carbonica, provided the personality type fits.

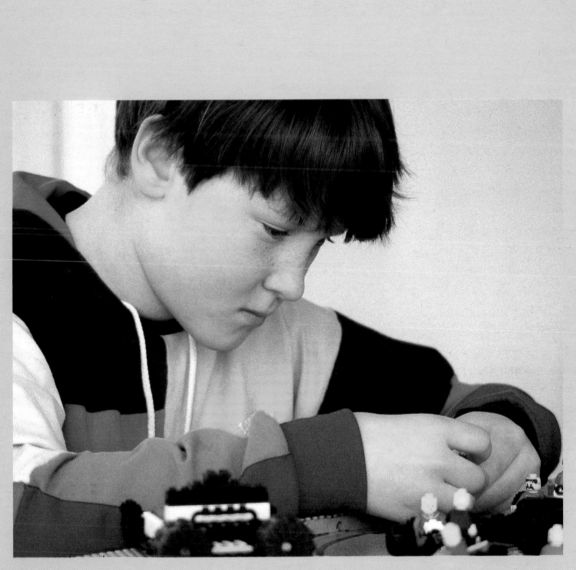

The Calcarea carbonica personality revels in tasks that involve patient, meticulous thoughts and actions, planned in a deliberate and step-by-step fashion. Trying to hurry and rush this type of child can bring out the stubborn streak.

IS YOUR CHILD A LYCOPODIUM TYPE?

Personality

A major feature of Lycopodium children is lack of self-confidence. Many of them are shy and timid, especially with people they do not know, or people with whom they do not feel comfortable.

Sometimes, however, the Lycopodium-type child tries to put on a cover-up act and become bossy, even dictatorial – with other children, and even with his or her own parents. But in unfamiliar situations, the child still wants the parents around for reassurance, just in case.

Fears and worries

Lycopodium children worry about how they will cope with public events, such as speaking in front of the school class, in case they make fools of themselves.

Often this worry is exaggerated, and to others, they seem to take themselves too seriously. But if a Lycopodium child feels a sense of failure, this can play havoc with his or her ego, which is usually rather brittle or frail.

Despite such fears, Lycopodium children often perform very well, once their initial inhibitions have been overcome. Since they are so unsure and lack confidence, they

---

> *Key Lycopodium features*
>
> • Shy, lacks confidence, anxious, worried
> • Fear of being seen to fail
> • Craving for sweets and sugary foods
> • Tendency to produce intestinal gases or wind

---

may try to compromise in order to avoid criticism or censure. This can lead to indecision. Or they may cry after being criticised or disciplined, due to their extreme sensitivity.

Typical fears of the Lycopodium child are the darkness or night-time and its associated bumps, noises, ghosts, and monsters, and also large animals such as horses and big dogs, as well as examinations, tests, and other situations where they might be "exposed" and seen as failures.

Physical features

The Lycopodium child is often slim, or even thin, and sometimes tall and rather gangling. The head can seem proportionally large compared with the body.

Babies and very young children may have an odd, wrinkly, adult-looking frown.

Likes and dislikes

Lycopodium children prefer to have their heads cool and their bodies warm. In the daily cycle of activity, they may have a quiet or low point in the late afternoon and early evening. Mornings are generally not popular, and they can wake up bad-tempered.

Lycopodium-type children should learn to avoid gassy foods, such as cabbages, beans, and onions, because these can cause uncomfortable flatulence. They much prefer sweet foods and warm drinks.

Symptoms and illnesses

* The stomach is usually a weak point. The Lycopodium type can suffer from wind and constipation, aggravated by anxiety and gassy foods.
* These digestive symptoms are often right-sided, or begin on the right side and move to the left.
* Colds and coughs may have a tendency to move down from the head and throat into the chest.
* As a constitutional remedy, all sorts of problems can be helped by Lycopodium, provided the personality type fits.

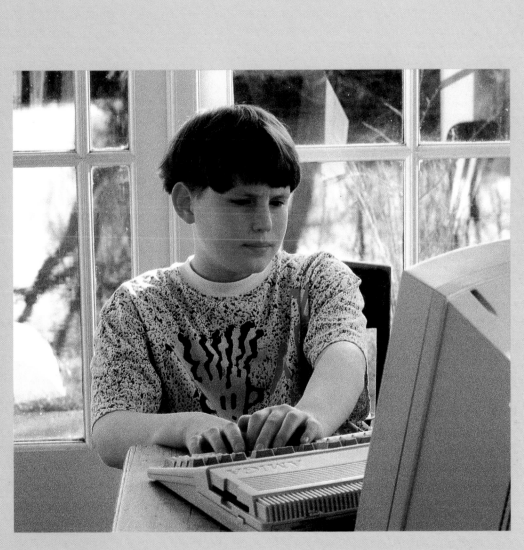

The Lycopodium constitution involves determination but also lack of self-confidence. This conflict can cause a fear of failure, which is covered up by being bossy and even arrogant.

IS YOUR CHILD A NAT MUR TYPE?

Personality

Natrum muriaticum (Nat mur) children tend to suffer from their basic over-sensitivity. It is the kind of sensitivity that is not on show, but which is private, and locked up deep inside.

So the Natrum muriaticum child may prefer to suffer and grieve alone, perhaps crying in his or her own room. Hurt feelings are not easily expressed to others, and the child fears being misunderstood and being laughed at.

On the outside, such children can appear to be very self-contained and independent. They also tend to be tidy and orderly. But the extreme sensitivity to the remarks and criticisms of others underlies almost everything they say and do.

Fears and worries

Natrum muriaticum children are self-conscious and worry about being the centre of attention. This is because they are so sensitive to the embarrassment caused by being told off or criticised – or even to being praised.

The Natrum muriaticum child may appear to be wise and responsible, way beyond her or his age. However deep inside, she

Key Nat mur features

• Very sensitive to comments and criticisms, however well meaning
• Suppressed or locked-up emotions that only show in private
• Wise and serious beyond her or his years
• Self-contained and independent

or he may be filled with sadness, guilt, and even resentment, that the most attentive parent may not suspect.

Natrum muriaticum children usually take emotional loss very much to heart. (Nat mur is one of the major homeopathic remedies for grief and sadness.)

In particular, they may worry about losses that are unlikely, and in any case beyond their control, like their parents or loved ones dying, or their pets passing away.

These children may also fear burglars and other intruders, and spiders.

Physical features

The Natrum muriaticum child is usually somewhat thin. He or she finds it difficult to put on weight, despite eating well.

Likes and dislikes

Natrum muriaticum children are uncomfortable in stuffy or warm places, and notably in hot sun, which can bring on headaches.

They may crave salt or salty things, and avoid fatty, greasy, or slimy foods. Ailments often become worse if they are at or near the sea.

Symptoms and illnesses

∗ Allergies and allergy-based problems, such as asthma and hayfever.
∗ A tendency to cold sores on and around the lips.
∗ Any discharges are often thin and watery, clear, or whitish.
∗ As a constitutional remedy, all sorts of problems can be helped by Natrum muriaticum, provided the personality type fits.

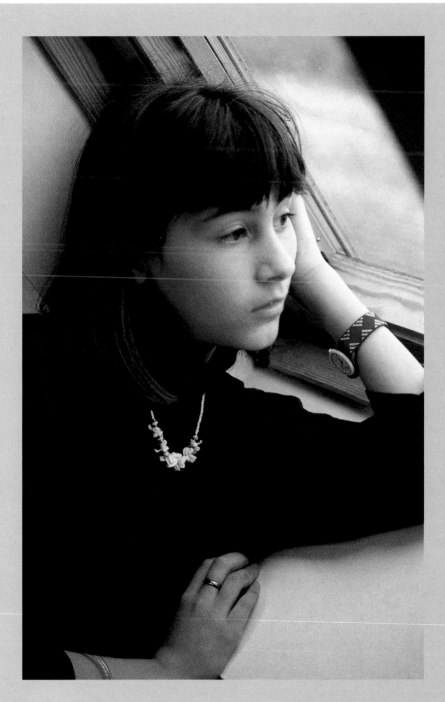

The Natrum muriaticum personality is essentially personal and private, introspective and possibly pessimistic. The child may dwell on and worry about what might go wrong – especially if it is out of his or her control.

IS YOUR CHILD A PHOSPHORUS TYPE?

Personality

Phosphorus children are generally warm-hearted, sympathetic, and affectionate. They love company and they also tend to attract it, because most people find their natural spontaneity, curiosity, and playful good nature very endearing. So they make friends quickly and easily, and they are open and honest about their problems and opinions.

The Phosphorus child often has a vivid imagination, and can be very creative. However he or she may become upset or even ill through over-excitement.

Fears and worries

These children require much attention and feedback from others, or they can become lonely and without an aim or focus.

If they are particularly highly strung, they can be nervous in the dark, from sudden noises, big bangs, or thunderstorms.

This need for attention, coupled with a loving personality, can cause the Phosphorus child to worry about the safety of his or her parents, friends, pets, or other loved ones. But he or she is seldom shy, and even when appearing so, the sparkling eyes

---

> *Key Phosphorus features*
>
> • Slightly delicate and fine looking
> • Warm, affectionate personality
> • Responds well to love and affection
> • May lack concentration and be easily distracted
> • Weak points include stomach, throat, and chest
> • Often of a nervous disposition

---

reveal the true friendly, outgoing aspects of the personality.

Physical features

The typical Phosphorus child is sometimes described as "delicate looking". This does not mean that he or she appears obviously ill or sick. It refers to a certain fineness or slenderness in build or stature, and in facial and other physical features.

The child is likely to be tall and slim, or perhaps truly thin, with good, clear skin, and long eyelashes.

Likes and dislikes

These children are often thirsty, and gulp down long, cold drinks. Unusually for many children, they are fond of spicy or salty foods, as well as ice cream (but then, which child is not fond of ice cream?).

They generally feel better when they are receiving attention, and particularly when they are being comforted and cuddled.

Symptoms and illnesses

* The stomach is sometimes a weak point. When the child is ill, he or she may vomit up cold food and drink, as soon as it has warmed up in the stomach.
* A greater tendency to diarrhoea than to constipation.
* Feelings of faintness and dizziness if blood sugar levels fall too low, so it is best for them not to miss meals.
* A tendency to nosebleeds.
* The chest can also be weak. So colds may easily go down to the chest, and laryngitis in the lower throat (larynx or voice-box) can progress to bronchitis in the lungs.
* As a constitutional remedy, all sorts of problems can be helped by Phosphorus, provided the personality type fits.

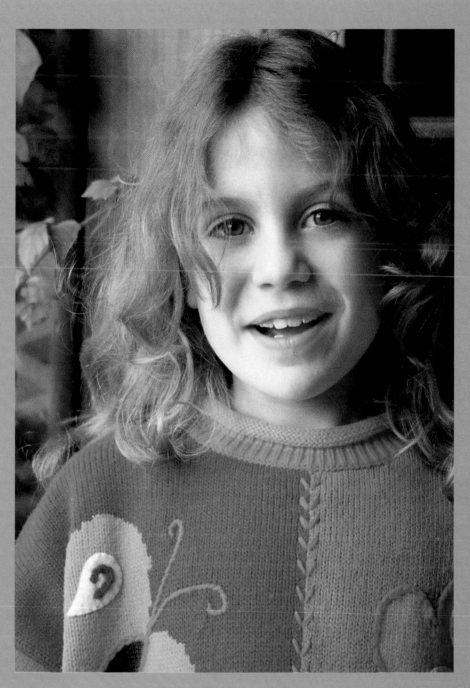

Everyone seems to love Phosphorus children, with their bright eyes and colourful nature. However, their high spirits may lead to illness, as they go "over the top" from too much excitement.

IS YOUR CHILD A PULSATILLA TYPE?

Personality

The biggest problem for Pulsatilla children is the fear of being alone or abandoned. So they tend to be timid, and avoid confrontation, and try to please – in fact, do anything to ensure that they are not rejected and left alone by their parents and friends.

This type of child is usually weepy and clinging under stress, and keeps close to parents in unfamiliar situations. Being told off or disciplined can be particularly painful.

Normally affectionate and loving by nature, the child is easily comforted by caring sympathy and a cuddle.

The moods of the Pulsatilla-type child are very changeable. Tears always seem to be near the surface, even when the child reaches an age when she or he should be growing out of such mood swings and becoming more mature and "grown up".

Indecision can be another problem. The typical Pulsatilla child would rather that someone else makes a decision, so that disagreements are avoided.

There is also a jealous side – especially where sibling rivalry is concerned.

Key Pulsatilla features

- Fear or worry of being abandoned
- Particularly sensitive to events such as changing school
- Indecisive and changeable, which includes moods, food preferences, and symptoms
- Delicate, shy appearance
- Prefers cool, fresh air

Fears and worries

As mentioned, the central fear is of being abandoned. The Pulsatilla child worries about any situation when this might occur. He or she is also likely to be very sensitive, and much affected by the loss of a friend, or by the trauma of life events such as moving house or changing school.

Physical features

Because of the very sensitive nature, the Pulsatilla constitution is more applicable to girls than boys. But it is by no means exclusively female.

The child may look sensitive, delicate, nervous, and shy, especially in mixed company. However, this is less noticeable in the company of parents or other familiar adults, when she or he looks and feels safe.

Likes and dislikes

The Pulsatilla child feels better when shown sympathy, and prefers cool, fresh air. She or he is not usually thirsty, and does not feel the cold too much.

There may be a dislike of rich, fatty foods, which can disagree and cause digestive upsets.

Symptoms and illnesses

* Pains and complaints tend to be changeable and shift from one area of the body to another – like the child's moods.

* These children are prone to earaches, colds that move down to the chest, and blocked noses.

* Any mucus is often yellow-green in colour.

* There is a susceptibility to recurring styes.

* As a constitutional remedy, all sorts of problems can be helped by Pulsatilla, provided the personality type fits. In particular, this remedy is best prescribed on the emotional state of mind, whatever the illness.

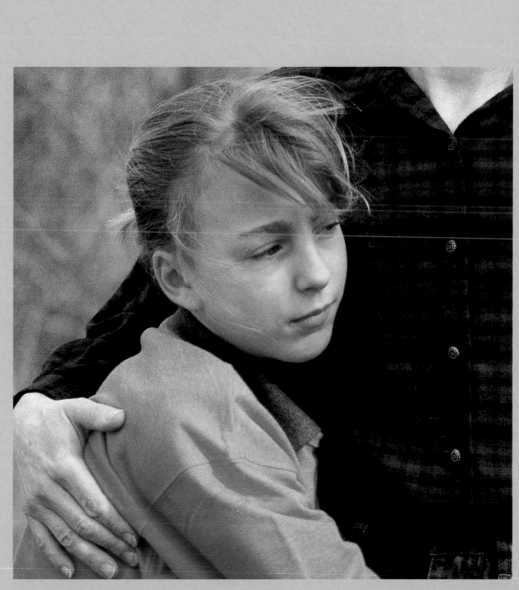

The Pulsatilla child may appear worried and clinging. She or he is comforted by warm sympathy, and a good cry to allow release of worry and tension.

IS YOUR CHILD A SULPHUR TYPE?

Personality

When Sulphur children are well, they are characteristically full of energy and curiosity. They are self confident and often stand out as natural leaders. Thinking quickly on their feet, they can readily put new information to practical use.

Most Sulphur-type children are extroverts. Some are even "loud-mouthed". A few are quieter, but even these still have great self confidence, perhaps with an annoying "know it all" manner.

They always seem to be asking questions, which can make their company quite exhausting. However, these children are also usually quick to learn, so their company is rewarding.

This type of child tends to be quite self-centred, and does not always notice what is going on around, if it is of no immediate interest or relevance. As a result, he or she can often appear insensitive, treading on the toes of more delicate friends.

The typical Sulphur child is usually untidy and lazy, and would slouch rather than stand upright. However he or she also tends to be good natured. When not procrastinating, this child can be very helpful, especially if given an opportunity to show off.

Key Sulphur features

- Confident, active, outgoing
- Sometimes self-centred and insensitive to the needs of others
- Physically big, strong, and boisterous
- Untidy, scruffy, even messy, in both appearance and habits
- Does not feel the cold

Fears and worries

In keeping with their confident and exuberant nature, not much frightens Sulphur-type children – except perhaps heights.

Physical features

The characteristic Sulphur physique is big and strong, although quieter types may be more slender. The child may be red faced and look rather untidy and scruffy, even unwashed.

Due to this mix of active and robust features, both physical and behavioural, the Sulphur type is probably more common among boys than girls.

Likes and dislikes

Sulphur types often dislike bathing and being washed, and they hate tidying their rooms!

They usually do not feel the cold and may stick their feet out of bed at night, to cool off. There is sometimes a low point at 11am, when the energy so important for this constitution runs low, so a snack can help.

There are tendencies to a sweet tooth, a liking for strongly flavoured foods, and a greater than average thirst.

Symptoms and illnesses

* In theory, almost any symptom or illness may strike. But the Sulphur constitution is strong, and so symptoms and ailments with underlying emotional causes may crop up less often.
* There may be an allergy to milk, which shows as digestive upsets such as vomiting or diarrhoea.
* There may also be allergy-based skin problems such as eczema, or other skin conditions.
* The skin tends to be very itchy.
* As a constitutional remedy, all sorts of problems can be helped by Sulphur, provided the personality type fits.

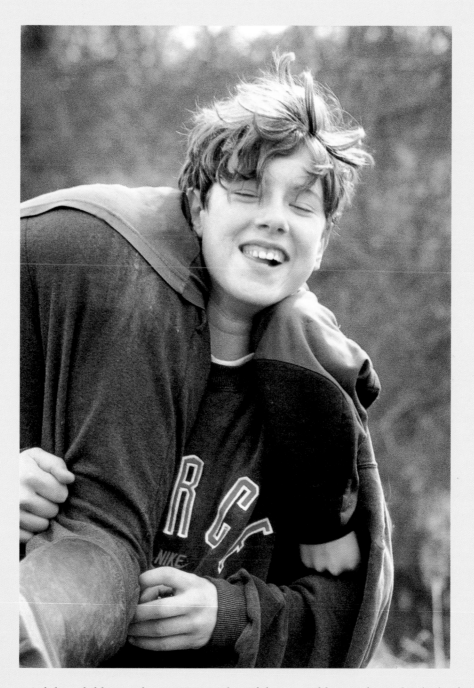

Sulphur children radiate energy and confidence, and love to be in the thick of the action. But they can also be lazy and they tend to put off what they dislike, such as having a wash or tidying the room.

Chapter Three

Treating Common Ailments

This chapter covers a number of problems which you can identify, prescribe for, and treat safely at home using homeopathy. With the aid of the relevant descriptions, most of the ailments lend themselves to self-diagnosis. However some, notably the children's diseases, should also receive the attention of a doctor.

It may seem strange, but in homeopathy, the precise name of the disease is not usually important. Most attention is paid to the symptom picture or pattern (see page 8).

Locating the ailment

When you feel you need to treat a problem with homeopathy, first consult the list of ailments and diseases (see The Common Ailments on page 53). These are grouped under seven main headings. You probably have some general idea of which ailment it might be. When you have located the appropriate page, check that the description and general symptom pattern fit your case. Then study the remedies to see which one is most suited to the detailed symptom pattern.

The modalities

Pay special attention to any mental or emotional signs and symptoms mentioned. Also take into account what homeopaths call the modalities. These are the factors that make the symptoms better or worse. You are now considering the individual person who is suffering,

"Homeopathy ... cures a larger percentage of cases than any other method of treatment and is beyond doubt safer, more economical, and the most complete medical science."

Mahatma Gandhi (1869-1948), Indian political and spiritual leader.

Natural minerals and rocks, such as chalk and flint, form the basis of many homeopathic remedies.

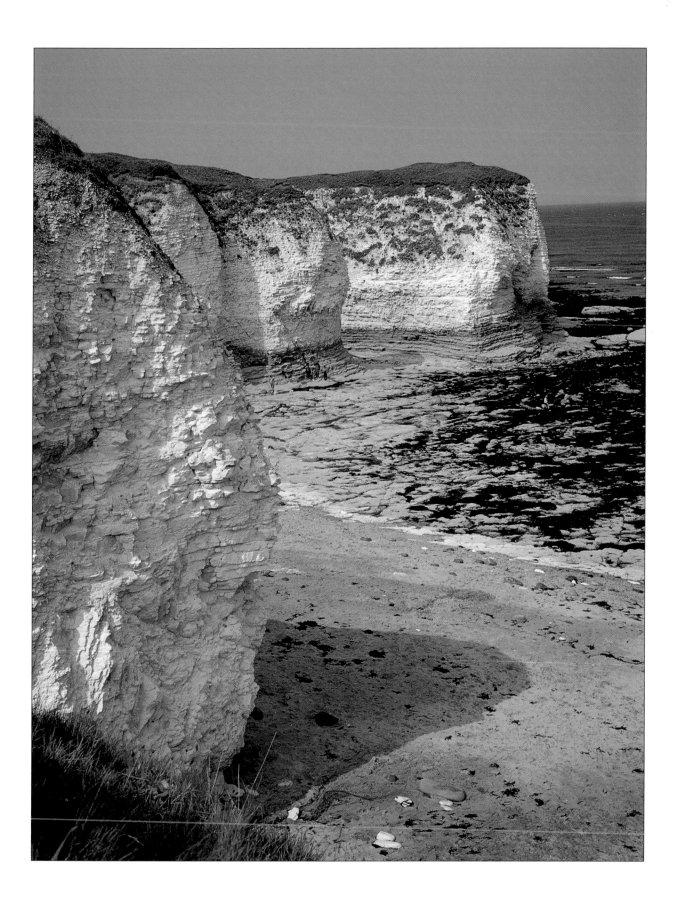

and not just the disease itself. So your chances of finding the right remedy and of curing the problem are greatly increased.

Check the remedy picture

When you have chosen the remedy, check its detailed description in Chapter Four, using the Index of Remedies (see page 99). This is a simplified, streamlined version of what homeopaths call the Materia Medica. If the information about the remedy seems to tie in with your case, and it all "feels" right to you, go ahead and give the appropriate dose according to the information below.

If the information does not seem to feel comfortable or right, you might like to return to the description of the ailment again. Check the other detailed symptom pictures under *Which remedy?*, and make your next most appropriate choice.

Wrong remedy?

Do not worry about giving or taking the wrong remedy (see page 17). You will not cause any harm, because of the minute amounts of ingredients in the pill. You can safely follow it with another remedy, which will hopefully be the right one.

Dose levels for non-urgent problems

Use only one remedy at a time, and only one pill of it at a time. It is very unwise to mix remedies or to give more than one pill simultaneously.

Ideally, you should take the remedy on a "clean tongue". That is, do not eat or drink anything for 15 minutes before or after the pill. This includes cleaning teeth and drinks. Generally, the pill should be sucked for about 30 seconds in the mouth. Then you can crunch it up and chew as you wish, before you swallow.

For general non-urgent situations, give one pill of the 30C potency each day (see page 14). Or give one pill of the 6C potency three times each day. Remember that one of the basic principles of homeopathy is that "less is more". In accordance with this principle, the higher the potency or dilution of a remedy, then the stronger, and deeper, and longer-lasting are its effects on the body.

Dose levels for urgent problems

In very acute or urgent situations, you can increase the frequency of the dose to one pill every hour, or even every 15 minutes. Do not worry about overdosing. Homeopathy is very safe. Even if a child swallows a whole handful of pills at once, by mistake or accident, no harm should be done.

In emergencies, too, do not worry about taking the remedy on a "clean tongue". The remedy should be used as quickly as possible, and it should work almost as well.

Handling and storing remedies

Handle only the remedy you are taking. If you touch others by accident, or drop the remedy you are using, throw away these pills at once. Do not put them back into the bottle.

Store remedies in a cool, dry place. Make sure that this is away from strong smells, bright lights, vibrations, and electromagnetic radiations. Also ensure that the pill bottle's top is securely tightened.

Interaction with other medical treatments

Homeopathy can be used safely with orthodox medical treatment – that is, the standard Western-type medicine. It should not interfere with medical drugs. However, the opposite may be a problem. Medical drugs can interfere with homeopathic treatments. It is advisable to consult your medical doctor before you stop or change the dose level of any course of medical drugs.

Homeopathy can also be used safely with most complementary or alternative forms of medicine and healing, including herbs and Bach flower remedies. However it is best to avoid any medicines and preparations containing camphor or eucalyptus. These can act as an antidote to homeopathic remedies, and work against their actions.

General precautions

• If you are in doubt about the identity of an illness, or the diagnosis does not seem to fit, consult a qualified medical doctor. This is especially important in the very young, the old, pregnant mothers, and those with a long-standing medical condition such as diabetes or epilepsy.

• In emergencies, homeopathy can be used in addition to orthodox treatments such as standard first aid techniques. However, always ensure you obtain appropriate emergency medical help before starting to use homeopathic remedies.

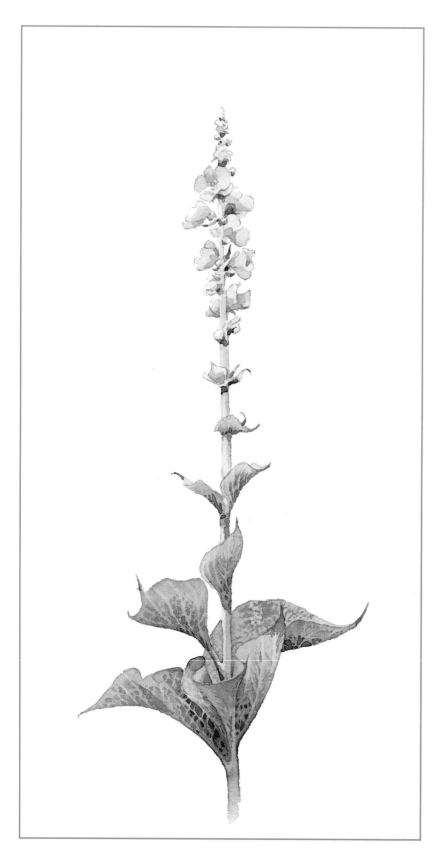

The remedy Verbascum is prepared from the common mullein plant. It is especially soothing for earaches, and is best applied in oil form, by inserting a few warmed drops of Verbascum oil into the ear.

The Common Ailments

Colds, Infections, and Fevers

Colds and influenza (flu)   55
Coughs and croup   56
Fevers   57
Sore throats and tonsillitis 58
Sinusitis   59

Digestive Problems

Diarrhoea   61
Indigestion   62
Nausea and vomiting   63
Haemorrhoids (piles)   64

Women's Problems

Cystitis   66
The menopause   66
Premenstrual tension (PMT)   67
Period pains   67
Anaemia   68
Mastitis and breastfeeding
  problems   68

Children's Problems

Asthma   70
Chickenpox   71
Colic   72
Croup   72
Earaches   73
Eczema   74
Rubella (German measles)   74
Emotional upsets   75
Measles   76
Mumps   77
Teething   77
Whooping cough   78

Allergies

Asthma   80
Hayfever   81

Emotional Strains and Stress

Anxiety and panic   83
Depression   84
Grief   84

Accidents, Emergencies, and Injuries

Bites and stings   86
Boils   86
Bruises   87
Burns   87
Cuts and sores   88
Eye injuries and strain   88
Eye inflammation   89
Styes   89
Fainting and collapse   90
Fractures   91
Nosebleeds   91
Shock   92
Sprains and strains   93
After surgery and dental
  treatment   93
Toothaches   94
Travel sickness   95

Colds, Infections, and Fevers

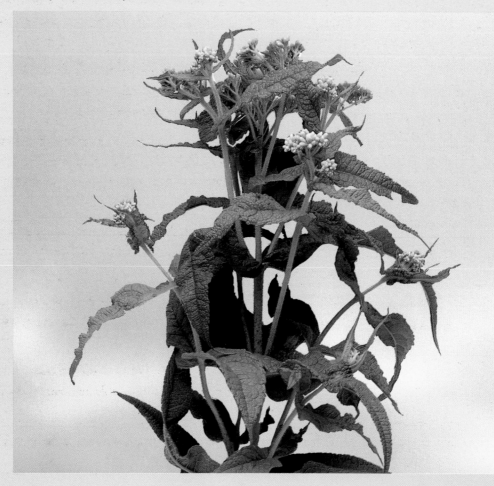

The body's powers of self-healing are usually sufficient to fight off a cold or soothe a fever within a few days. Homeopathic remedies can help to ease symptoms, and also shorten the illness by assisting the body's fight-back. The remedy Eupatorium, prepared from the herb boneset (above), is especially suited in influenza, when one of the main symptoms is aching bones.

COLDS AND INFLUENZA (FLU)

Causes

The common cold is caused by a virus called the rhinovirus. This regularly changes, or mutates, so the body cannot build up resistance or immunity to it. Flu is also a viral illness.

Symptoms

It is sometimes difficult to know when the runny or stuffy nose, sore eyes, and tickly throat of a bad cold, have been joined by the higher fever (39°C, 102°F) and vaguely aching joints of mild influenza. From a homeopathic point of view this is unimportant, since the remedies are much the same. A healthy body should conquer a cold in a few days. If you do not feel better, or if the symptoms seem to be progressing towards flu, a remedy can help to boost your body's defences.

✓ Prompt rest with plenty of warm drinks is often the best remedy. Too many people try to "work through" a cold, and end up feeling worse.

✓ If flu strikes, go to bed and rest, keeping the room warm but also well ventilated.

✓ If you get more than two or three colds each year, your immune system may benefit from being strengthened. Consult a homeopath.

Which remedy?

● If the symptoms strike suddenly, particularly at night or after exposure to cold dry winds, and you are thirsty, feverish, and sweaty, and still in the early stages of the illness, choose ☞ *Aconite.*

● When you are still in the early stages of the illness, with no prominent symptoms apart from feeling generally run down, and perhaps some thirst, choose ☞ *Ferrum phos.*

● If the cold starts in your nose with a watery yet burning discharge, and you sneeze frequently and feel chilly and restless, and you want sips of water, and then the cold threatens to go down into your chest, choose ☞ *Arsenicum.*

● When your nose runs with a burning discharge, and your eyes are sore and smarting and also runny, but the tears are weak and watery, choose ☞ *Allium cepa.*

● When the fever increases, and you suddenly develop a red burning face and throbbing headache, yet your skin is dry and you are not thirsty, choose ☞ *Belladonna.*

● If your symptoms develop slowly, and you feel extremely thirsty for long drinks of cold water, and you are irritable and want to be left alone and quiet, choose ☞ *Bryonia.*

● After the cold has gone to your chest, producing a dry painful cough, choose ☞ *Bryonia.*

● If your main symptoms are shivers and shakes, and you feel very tired and weak with heavy muscles, with perhaps a headache and a slight thirst, choose ☞ *Gelsemium.*

● Should the cold develop into influenza and get "into your bones" so that they ache, and you feel thirsty, but your symptoms (apart from the headache) improve as you sweat, choose ☞ *Eupatorium.*

COUGHS AND CROUP

Cough causes and symptoms

Coughs have various causes and many forms. They may be due to infection, to impure air, or to irritation by hard swallowed items such as fish bones. The many varieties of coughs include soft or harsh, dry or productive, irritating or relieving. Consider the type of cough carefully, in order to select the most suitable remedy.

Croup

Croup is an extremely harsh-sounding, persistent cough that affects mainly small children. Remedies for adults are described here. Croup in children is covered in more detail on page 72.

✓ Most healthy people can shake off a cough in a few days. If the problem continues, or if the cough worsens, a remedy may help the natural healing processes to overcome the cause.

✓ Rest in a warm but well-aired place. Too much warmth and stuffiness can aggravate a cough – as can cold draughts.

✓ A moist atmosphere, produced by steam from a gently warmed saucepan, can ease an aggravating cough.

✓ If a child suffers a bad attack of croup, and has difficulty breathing, get medical help or advice urgently (see page 72).

Which remedy?

● For a cough that is hoarse, dry, and painful, and so forceful – especially at night – that it makes you pant or even takes your breath away, choose ☞ *Aconite*.

● If your cough is hard, dry, and painful, and hurts your chest so much that you have to hold your ribs, and you thirst for long drinks of cold water, and you feel better when sitting upright but worse in a warm room, choose ☞ *Bryonia*.

● If your cough is so incessant and barking that it makes you breathless and almost retch, and you hold the sides of your abdomen to ease the pain, and your throat seems tickled as though by a feather, choose ☞ *Drosera*.

● When your cough is painful and barking, and worsens in cold air or when you are cold, and your chest rattles with thick yellow mucus that is hard to bring up, and you feel weak and bad tempered, choose ☞ *Hepar sulph*.

● For a tickling throat and cough brought on by breathing fresh air, and when your chest hurts, and you bring up copious frothy sputum (phlegm), yet you prefer to cover your mouth, choose ☞ *Rumex*.

● If your hollow barking cough sounds like sawing wood, and you feel suffocated because your chest seems so full, choose ☞ *Spongia*.

● If the symptoms of croup are present, including wheezy breathing and a harsh hollow cough that comes in tiring attacks, usually at night, there are three main remedies. First choose ☞ *Aconite*.

● If Aconite does not help croup after a few hours, choose ☞ *Spongia*.

● If Spongia is also unsuccessful for croup, choose ☞ *Hepar sulph*.

FEVERS

How high is a fever?

A fever is an increase in body temperature above the normal 37°C (98.4°F). A mild fever is 38-39°C (100-102°F), and shows that the body is fighting the illness. A high fever is 40°C (104°F) or above, and requires urgent medical advice.

Fevers and other symptoms

The remedies suggested here are useful when the fever is the primary symptom. The secondary symptoms guide you to the most suitable remedy. When a fever is one of the secondary symptoms, consult the pages dealing with the main symptom, such as a cough.

✓ A fever, in itself, is nothing to be concerned about. However if it rises to 40°C (104°F) or above, the body's temperature control mechanism may become over-stretched. Urgent action is necessary.

✓ There are many ways to cool the body. Wear light clothing, wipe the face and arms with a cool sponge or flannel, and take plenty of long, cooling drinks.

✓ If a sudden fever is accompanied by an intense headache and/or neck pain, consult a doctor urgently. Do likewise if your temperature does not return to normal after a couple of days, or if you feel worried.

Which remedy?

● For a relatively uncomplicated mild fever, with perhaps a modest thirst, choose ☞ *Ferrum phos.*

● If the fever came on suddenly, especially at night, and you are thirsty and sweaty, choose ☞ *Aconite.*

● If you feel feverish and restless, and you long for cool flowing air, and your glands are tender and swollen, but you are not thirsty, choose ☞ *Apis.*

● When you feel very chilly, anxious, and restless, and you want frequent sips of water, and you may be wheezing and sneezing with a head cold, choose ☞ *Arsenicum.*

● For the fever that comes on suddenly, usually at night, and seems centred in the head where it causes a throbbing headache and red face, yet there is little thirst or sweating, choose ☞ *Belladonna.*

● If your temperature rises slowly, and you long for drinks of cold water, and you are irritable and want to be left alone, choose ☞ *Bryonia.*

● When the fever makes you shiver and tremble, and you feel weak with aching muscles, but you are not very thirsty, choose ☞ *Gelsemium.*

● If your glands are swollen, and you are thirsty and sweaty and irritable, and you have bad breath and lots of saliva, with the fever possibly rising and falling, choose ☞ *Mercurius.*

● When cool fresh air makes you feel better, and you are not particularly thirsty, and perhaps you feel weepy and lonely, choose ☞ *Pulsatilla.*

● If the fever seems to burn, yet there is a chill especially down your back, and perhaps you crave ice-cold water, choose ☞ *Phosphorus.*

● For the fever that makes you restless and chilly, and you feel worse if you remove any clothes or bedcovers, choose ☞ *Rhus tox.*

SORE THROATS AND TONSILLITIS

Causes

Sore throats can result from either viral or bacterial infection. They usually clear up without treatment, but homeopathic remedies can help speed healing.

Symptoms

The usual symptoms are throat pain that worsens on swallowing, hoarseness, and inability to clear the throat. Tonsillitis is redness and swelling of the palatine tonsils, two small bumps at the very back of the throat. They can become painfully enlarged, usually as a result of infection. There are many gradations between sore throats and full-blown tonsillitis.

✓ Most cases of sore throats and tonsillitis heal over a few days, especially with homeopathy. But seek help if the problem persists for more than three or four days. You could have a stubborn bacterial infection sometimes known as a "strep throat" (caused by *Streptococcus* bacteria).

✓ If you get more than two or three attacks of sore throats in a year, your immune system may be weakened. Consider a visit to a homeopath for constitutional treatment.

✓ Gargle every hour or two with warm, weak salt water to reduce the soreness.

Which remedy?

● If your symptoms appear suddenly, usually at night after getting a chill, and your throat feels hot and dry, you are thirsty, and swallowing is painful, choose ☞ *Aconite*.

● If your throat looks red and puffy, and although you are not thirsty, the stinging pain is helped by cool drinks, choose ☞ *Apis*.

● When your throat feels very sore (as if a fish bone is sticking in it), you cough up green mucus, and you feel bad-tempered and chilly, choose ☞ *Hepar sulph*.

● For throat soreness that is on the left, or moves from left to right, and which may extend to the ear, and – strangely – when swallowing liquids you have a feeling of lumps in the throat, which you cannot bear to be touched or constricted, choose ☞ *Lachesis*.

● If the pain is on the right or moves from right to left, and improves with warm drinks, but possibly worsens in the late afternoon or early evening, choose ☞ *Lycopodium*.

● When your breath smells and you have profuse, yellow, slimy saliva, and you are sweaty and thirsty, with a raw throat and a swollen flabby tongue, choose ☞ *Mercurius*.

● If your throat looks dark or bluish-red inside, and the pain feels like a hot lump, and it hurts even more when you swallow, choose ☞ *Phytolacca*.

● When symptoms come on suddenly with little or no thirst, and you have a high temperature, a red face and your eye pupils look wide open, and your tonsils appear bright red and they throb painfully, choose ☞ *Belladonna*.

SINUSITIS

Causes

The sinuses are small cavities in the skull bones, around the eyes and above the nose. In sinusitis, the membranes lining the cavities become swollen and sore, usually due to infection by bacteria.

Symptoms

The main symptoms are a blocked nose, nasal discharge, frontal headaches or facial pains, and perhaps a fever. Colds or allergic reactions may set off the inflammation.

✓ Avoid hot, stuffy places. Try to stay in cool surroundings with a flow of fresh air.

✓ Every two or three hours, inhale warm, humid, steamy air to loosen and liquefy the mucus. But avoid menthol, eucalyptus, or camphor preparations, since these can counteract homeopathic remedies.

✓ Try different positions for resting your head, so that the affected sinuses do not become clogged with mucus and more inflamed.

Which remedy?

● If, in addition to the usual symptoms, you are sweaty and thirsty, with bad breath and yellow-green nasal mucus, choose ☞ *Mercurius*.

● If you have the usual symptoms, and in addition there is a thick yellow-green nasal discharge, and you have little or no thirst, and you feel better in fresh cool air, choose ☞ *Pulsatilla*.

● When you have the symptoms of sinusitis, and in addition shivering, weakness, and an ache at the back of the head, choose ☞ *Gelsemium*.

● For sinusitis that produces a lot of yellow-green mucus in the nose, and also your neck glands may be swollen, and perhaps the symptoms have dragged on for several days, choose ☞ *Silica*.

● For sinusitis that is worse in the late afternoon and early evening, and worse on the right side of the face, choose ☞ *Lycopodium*.

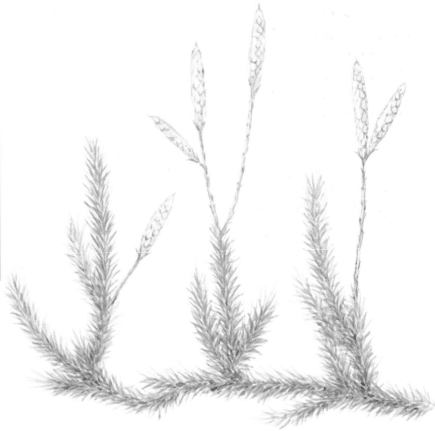

Lycopodium is a useful remedy for a sore throat or sinusitis, when the symptoms are worse on the right side.

Digestive Problems

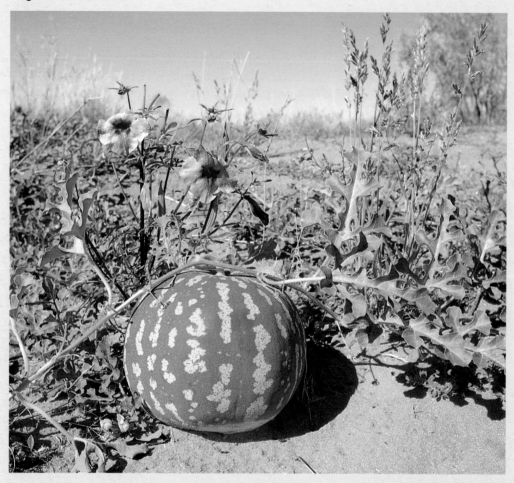

In the past, many digestive upsets were caused by germs on infected foods. Today most foods are safer to eat. Yet digestive problems still occur, often stemming from unsuitable diets or sensitivity to certain chemicals in foods. The remedy Colocynthis, from the bitter cucumber plant, has soothing effects on the digestive system when agonizing, cramping pain is involved.

DIARRHOEA

Causes

Diarrhoea has many causes, from eating contaminated food, to food allergy, to extreme fright! However, you may have to accept that in certain cases, there is no clear cause.

Course of action

In general, diarrhoea is the body's natural way of quickly removing impurities and toxins from the digestive system. For this reason, it is best not to interfere with the process straight away. Follow the self-help recommendations below. If the problem has not improved in 6-8 hours, try a remedy.

✓ Like vomiting (see page 63), diarrhoea can cause dehydration and loss of body minerals. Prevent this by drinking plenty of water or very weak fruit juices. Avoid strong, concentrated juices.

✓ The more you rest, the quicker the problem should clear.

✓ As you recover, eat small amounts of bland foods such as bread, pasta, or rice.

✓ If copious diarrhoea continues for more than 24 hours, or 12 hours in a baby or infant, obtain medical advice.

✓ These remedies may be useful on holiday, when unusual food or water can easily upset your stomach.

Which remedy?

● If you feel chilly, weak, and restless, and you perhaps have nausea and vomiting with the diarrhoea, choose ☞ *Arsenicum.*

● For diarrhoea that is accompanied by agonising stomach cramps, as if your guts are being squeezed, but which is eased by bending double or by hard pressure on the area, and you feel anger, choose ☞ *Colocynthis.*

● If the diarrhoea is painless but very watery, as if running from a tap, and you crave cold water which you vomit up as soon as it has warmed in your stomach, choose ☞ *Phosphorus.*

● When the diarrhoea is putrid but expelled painlessly in a gushing torrent, and you cannot bear any thought of food or drink, choose ☞ *Podophyllum.*

● If you have diarrhoea and also violent vomiting, along with sweats, coldness, and painful cramps, and you crave ice-cold water, choose ☞ *Veratrum album.*

● If the diarrhoea is brought on by anxiety, worry, anticipation, or excitement, choose ☞ *Arg nit.*

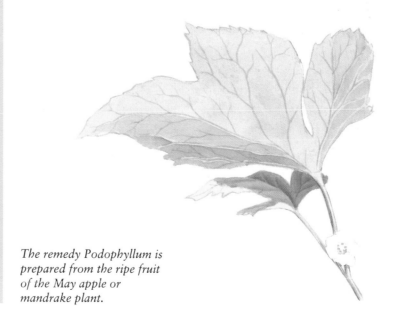

The remedy Podophyllum is prepared from the ripe fruit of the May apple or mandrake plant.

INDIGESTION

Causes

The causes of indigestion are very varied, from eating or drinking too much or too fast, to taking meals at unaccustomed times, to eating certain foods which disagree with you.

Symptoms and actions

The main symptoms include heartburn, wind (gas), cramping pains in the abdomen, hiccups, and occasionally nausea.

The stomach, intestines, and other digestive parts usually sort out the problem themselves, but the following two remedies often help in prolonged cases.

If the main symptoms are diarrhoea or nausea, or for colic in babies and children, see the appropriate pages.

✓ If the indigestion persists and becomes localized in the lower right abdomen, or if it is accompanied by fever, seek urgent medical advice.

✓ If the abdomen goes hard and "stiff" like a board, obtain medical help, in case of peritonitis.

Which remedy?

● If you have a general or recurring weakness in the digestive system, perhaps triggered by anxiety or by eating flatulent foods such as cabbages or beans, choose ☞ *Lycopodium*.

● If you are prone to indigestion because of indulging in rich foods and drinks, and the food sits like an immovable load in your stomach, choose ☞ *Nux vomica*.

● If the indigestion is linked to a hangover headache, due to drinking too much alcohol, choose ☞ *Nux vomica*.

Nux vomica is made from the seeds of the poison-nut tree. It is both a first-aid remedy and a long-term treatment for many digestive and other problems.

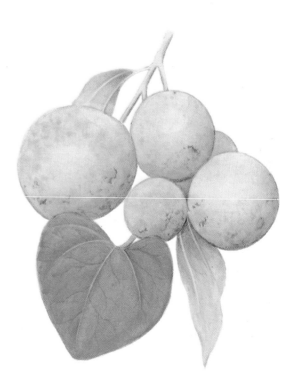

NAUSEA AND VOMITING

Causes and symptoms

Vomiting is a natural way for the body to clear out its digestive system, in the quickest possible way. Nausea is usually a warning that this is going to happen, but it can indicate other ailments, such as an ear infection that interferes with balance and brings on dizziness and giddiness.

Vomiting is usually caused by an infection that has got into the stomach or intestines, perhaps brought on by food poisoning. It can also be due to food allergy.

Course of action

No action is needed if the vomiting and nausea clear up in a few hours and you feel better. But if it persists, try one of these remedies to "break" the problem.

✓ Like diarrhoea (see page 61), vomiting can cause dehydration. Take water regularly in small sips, if your body tolerates it.

✓ If the vomiting has not lessened after 8-10 hours, seek medical help, especially if a child is involved.

✓ If the vomiting is accompanied by a headache and/or neck pain, get urgent medical help.

✓ These remedies may be useful on holiday, when unusual food or water can easily upset your stomach.

Which remedy?

● If the vomiting is accompanied by diarrhoea and stomach pains, and you feel weak, chilly and restless, and you wish to take sips of cold water but cannot keep them down, choose ☞ *Arsenicum.*

● If Arsenicum does not work, and you still have the above symptoms, and your stomach feels hollow and empty, choose ☞ *Phosphorus.*

● When the stomach pains make you want to lie alone and still on the side that hurts, and you feel very thirsty and want lots of cold water, choose ☞ *Bryonia.*

● For vomiting accompanied by stomach pains, that are eased only by bending double or pressing hard on the painful part, choose ☞ *Colocynthis.*

● If vomiting does not lessen your nausea or make you feel better, but your tongue remains clean and uncoated, choose ☞ *Ipecac.*

● If you feel greatly nauseous but you cannot bring up much, and you feel irritable and chilly, and the food lies like a heavy load in your stomach, choose ☞ *Nux vomica.*

● If you start vomiting after catching a chill and you have become feverish, choose ☞ *Eupatorium.*

● When the vomiting is particularly violent, and you also have diarrhoea, you feel cold and sweaty, and you want drinks of ice-cold water, choose ☞ *Veratrum album.*

HAEMORRHOIDS (PILES)

Causes

Haemorrhoids are a common problem. They are varicose veins (swollen, engorged blood vessels) around the anus or back passage. Sometimes they develop for no obvious reason. In other cases they may be due to straining very hard to pass hard stools, as a consequence of a low-fibre diet.

Symptoms

Haemorrhoids vary in severity from itchy, to uncomfortable, to very painful. They may remain inside the rectal and anal passages, or protrude from the anal opening. They may rupture when stools are passed, causing a bloody discharge. These remedies can help in mild cases.

✓ Check that your diet is well balanced, with plenty of fresh fruits and vegetables, and other high-fibre foods. This makes the digestion more efficient and the stools softer and easily passed.

✓ If these remedies do not help, consult a homeopath, who may prescribe a remedy according to your personality and constitution (see page 32).

✓ If you pass blood often, or if your stools are black with congealed blood, seek prompt medical help. The problem may not be haemorrhoids, and also there is a risk of anaemia.

Which remedy?

● If the haemorrhoids cause a burning pain, and visibly protrude like a bunch of grapes, and a sharp pain shoots up your back, choose ☞ *Aesculus*. This is usually applied as a purpose-made cream or lotion directly to the area.

● If the haemorrhoids are very bruised and sore, and they feel as though they might burst, choose ☞ *Hamamelis*. This is usually applied as a purpose-made cream or lotion directly to the area.

● For haemorrhoids that itch, and are exacerbated by too much straining during bowel movements, and the stools are unsatisfactory as though not all of them have been passed, choose ☞ *Nux vomica*. Take this as a homeopathic pill in the normal way.

● If the haemorrhoids seem to have become an almost permanent fixture, and they burn and smart with pain, and you are prone to diarrhoea early in the morning, choose ☞ *Sulphur*. Take this as a homeopathic pill in the normal way.

The fresh bark of the plant commonly known as witch hazel is the source of the remedy Hamamelis.

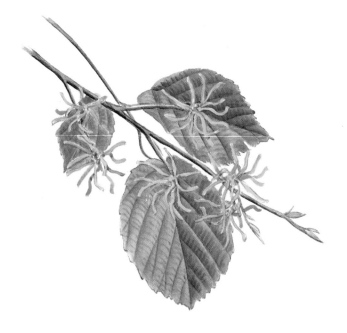

Women's Problems

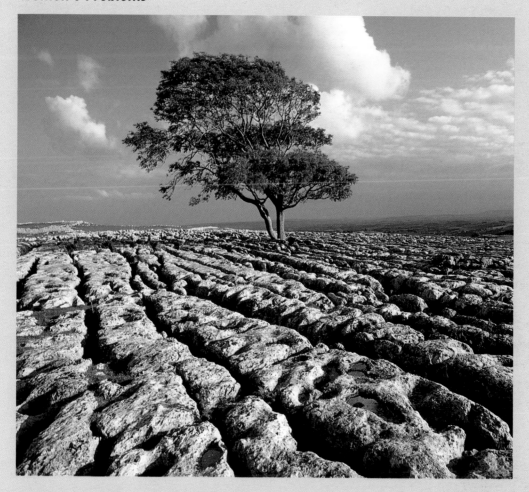

Homeopathy can be gentle, yet powerful, in the treatment of women's problems. These include difficulties with the "stages of life" and also with infections and inflammations, such as cystitis. The remedy Calcarea carbonica, which is chalk or lime (a mineral common in limestone landscapes, above) can be very effective in promoting the production of breast milk in nursing mothers.

CYSTITIS

Causes and symptoms

Cystitis is a sore and inflamed bladder lining, usually caused by infection. The main symptoms are burning pains during urination and a strong need, not always successful, to pass urine.

✓ Take extra care with hygiene.

✓ Drink plenty of water to flush out the kidneys and bladder.

✓ Consult a homeopath if the cystitis recurs. A remedy may help to strengthen your immune system.

✓ If cystitis persists for more than a few days, consult your doctor.

Which remedy?

● If you feel a desperate urge to urinate but hardly any urine is passed, the urine feels almost scalding, and the pain is intense, choose ☞ *Cantharis*. (This is the usual first remedy.)

● If the urine feels burning, and you pass a little by accident when you cough, choose ☞ *Causticum*.

● When the usual symptoms are present, and the pain is worse when you finish urinating, choose ☞ *Sarsaparilla*.

● For long-term or persistent cystitis, which is made worse by sexual intercourse (sometimes called "honeymoon cystitis"), choose ☞ *Staphysagria*.

THE MENOPAUSE

Causes and symptoms

The menopause is when the menstrual periods stop, usually in the late forties or early fifties. It is a perfectly natural process. Remedies can help associated problems such as night sweats and hot flushes.

✓ Symptoms usually last only a few months. If they persist or become severe, see a homeopath or doctor.

✓ Listen to the advice of valued friends and family members. They may have a different viewpoint.

Which remedy?

● If your moods and emotions swing from one extreme to the other, and you have hot flushes that rise up your body towards your head, choose ☞ *Lachesis*.

● When you are very weepy, feeling emotionally sad and alone, and even seemingly in despair, choose ☞ *Pulsatilla*.

● If you become very irritable, and you lose interest in your family and friends, even though they are very dear to you, and you have sweating and hot flushes, choose ☞ *Sepia*.

PREMENSTRUAL TENSION (PMT)

Causes and symptoms

The symptoms of PMT (also called premenstrual syndrome, PMS) usually come on about a week before the start of the menstrual period. They can range from utter despair, through weepy sadness, to irritability, and even violent rage. The effects generally fade as the period begins, although they can persist into the next cycle ("post-menstrual tension").

Which remedy?

● If your main emotions are jealousy and suspicion, and you are usually very talkative and passionate by nature, choose ☞ *Lachesis.*

● When you are tearful and sad, or perhaps you feel sad but cannot cry at all, and you want to be left alone to keep all your feelings to yourself, choose ☞ **Natrum muriaticum.**

● If you are very weepy, and you feel alone and abandoned and unsupported, and you feel better in company and worse in a stuffy room, choose ☞ **Pulsatilla.**

● For total indifference and lack of interest, even towards your loved ones, and you are bad-tempered and touchy, choose ☞ *Sepia.*

PERIOD PAINS

Symptoms

Many women experience cramps or aches in the lower abdomen, during the menstrual period. These are usually worse on the first few days, and then fade.

The venomous bushmaster, a type of pit viper from tropical America, is the source of the remedy Lachesis.

✓ The application of warmth from a towel-wrapped hot water bottle, or a soothing massage, may help.

✓ If the pains become unbearable, and especially if accompanied by a heavier than usual blood loss, obtain medical advice.

Which remedy?

● When the pain is only eased when you bend double or press the site hard, and you also feel extremely irritable, choose ☞ *Colocynthis.*

● If the pain comes on before the period, and is worse on the left side, and you cannot bear any touch or pressure on this painful part, yet the pain ceases as soon as the blood flow starts, choose ☞ *Lachesis.*

● For shooting pains that improve with warmth or gentle massage, choose ☞ **Mag phos.**

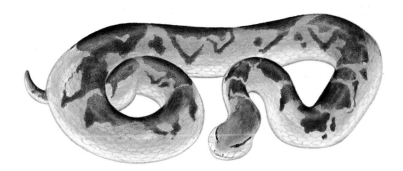

ANAEMIA

Causes and symptoms

Anaemia is a deficiency of the blood's oxygen-carrying ability, usually caused by lack of iron. The main symptoms are paleness, fatigue, panting on exertion, heart palpitations, and digestive disturbances. It is more common in women because of the demands of menstruation and pregnancy.

✓ Eat foods rich in iron, such as liver, egg yolk, shellfish, parsley, wholewheat bread, and green vegetables.

Which remedy?

● Take the homeopathic remedy *Ferrum phos* daily, for several months if necessary. This is the major remedy for anaemia where there is iron deficiency. Discontinue it when your health returns to normal.

✓ Anaemia may have other causes besides iron deficiency. If it persists, consult your doctor for an examination and blood tests.

MASTITIS AND BREASTFEEDING PROBLEMS

Causes and symptoms

Mastitis is inflammation of the breast, usually due to bacterial infection. It is most common when breastfeeding, because germs spread from the nipple along the milk ducts into the breast tissue, and the ducts then become blocked.

✓ If you become suspicious about any swelling or lump in the breast, especially if it is painless, always consult your doctor without delay.

Which remedy?

● If the breast is red and hot and throbs painfully, and perhaps has red streaks radiating from the nipple area, choose ☞ *Belladonna.*

● When the breast feels hard, heavy, and painful, and there may be an associated headache, choose ☞ *Bryonia.*

● When the breast feels heavy and "stony" with hard nodes, and is also very swollen and tender, and the nipple is cracked and sensitive, making breastfeeding painful, choose ☞ *Phytolacca.*

● If breastfeeding is difficult because there is not enough milk, choose ☞ *Calcarea carbonica.*

● When there may be an emotional cause linked to the mastitis or milk shortage, and you feel weepy and lacking support, choose ☞ *Pulsatilla.*

Children's Problems

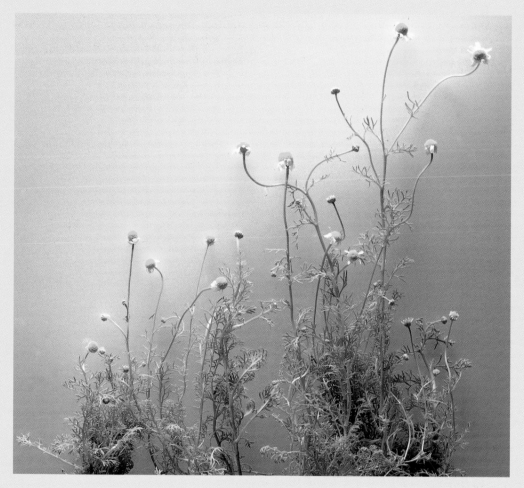

Children are especially responsive to homeopathic remedies such as Chamomilla, prepared from the herb chamomile (above). If the symptom picture is not clear, or the remedy seems ineffective, try prescribing from the constitutional type of the child when healthy, rather than from the current illness (see page 32).

ASTHMA

Causes and symptoms

The causes and effects of asthma are described in the Allergy section (see page 80). The chief symptom is difficult, wheezy breathing.

How common?

Recent years have seen something of an epidemic of asthma in children. It is rapidly becoming more common – in some regions more than one in ten children under the age of 12 years are affected. It can develop at any age, and may be linked to other allergy-based conditions such as eczema (see page 74).

✓ Follow the general self-help advice for asthma on page 80.

✓ Severe attacks of asthma are frightening, especially for children, and can be dangerous. Try to remain calm, and transmit this to the child.

✓ Get medical help immediately if you have not been told what to do.

✓ If your child suffers from asthma, consult a homeopath. Many cases respond very well to homeopathic remedies.

✓ As with eczema (see page 74), the most natural and satisfactory way to treat asthma is to strengthen your child's immune system. Consult a homeopath, but be aware that such treatment takes time.

Which remedy?

The following remedies are suitable for easing mild attacks. If the child becomes extremely breathless and the usual measures are having no effect, obtain emergency medical help.

● When attacks tend to occur at night (12pm-3am), and the child feels better when sitting up or walking around, and he or she may become tired or even exhausted after the attack, choose ☞ *Arsenicum*.

● If the child feels particularly irritable or even angry during an attack, choose ☞ *Chamomilla*.

● Should tension, irritation, or outright anger seem to trigger the attack, choose ☞ *Chamomilla*.

● If the child feels nauseous, and the chest seems full of mucus that he or she cannot cough up, and the child feels better in fresh air, choose ☞ *Ipecac*.

● If the child is normally affectionate and dependent, and the attacks make him or her feel worse when in a hot stuffy room, but the attacks are eased by cool fresh air, choose ☞ *Pulsatilla*.

● If the attacks are triggered by damp, or wet weather, or a cold, or exertion, and they tend to happen in the early hours of the morning, choose ☞ *Nat sulph*.

CHICKENPOX

Causes and symptoms

This is a common childhood infection, especially in very young children. The same virus that causes chickenpox is, in adult life, responsible for shingles – a painful skin eruption that affects the nerves. So these remedies could also be useful for shingles.

Chickenpox usually starts with a fever and a rash over most of the body. The spots become deep red, then turn to small blisters. These fill with pus, come to a head, and form scabs. The scabs dry and shrink and fall off, as the skin slowly heals. The whole illness lasts about two weeks. The main problems are itchiness of the spots and scabs, and the scars which may be left if these are picked or scratched.

✓ Chickenpox is seldom serious, but it is contagious until all the pustules (the pox) have turned to scabs.

✓ Soothing ointments or balms such as Calendula cream or moisturizing cream help to ease the itching. Use these only after the spots have come to a head.

✓ It may be difficult, but discourage the child from scratching the spots. This can cause skin scarring which may be permanent. For babies and young children, use woollen mittens to prevent scratching.

Which remedy?

● If the rash develops very slowly, the spots are full of pus, and the child is sleepy and perhaps has a cough, choose ☞ *Ant tart*.

● For the child with a high temperature, a red face, a throbbing headache, and a hot dry skin, choose ☞ *Belladonna*. (Belladonna is best used at the beginning of the disease.)

● If the spots become infected and turn septic, and the child is sweaty and thirsty, and he or she becomes considerably worse at night, choose ☞ *Mercurius*.

● If the child becomes emotional, weeping, and clinging, and he or she feels better when in cool fresh air, choose ☞ *Pulsatilla*.

● If the child is extremely restless, and the itching is so intense that he or she cannot stop scratching, which leads to great distress, choose ☞ *Rhus tox*.

The remedy Antimonium tartaricum is based on substances from the tartrate group. Tartrates are common in many fruits, especially grapes.

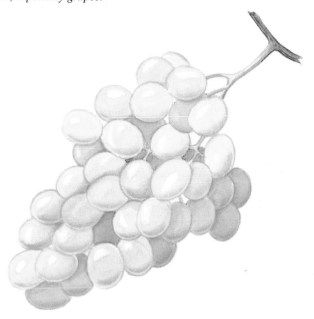

COLIC

Causes and symptoms

Colic is a common problem in small babies. It is a form of indigestion (see page 62) – a digestive upset causing wind and sharp spasms of abdominal pain.

✓ Colic often occurs at the same time each day, such as in the evening, when the parents are also tired.

✓ Since babies and small children cannot explain their symptoms, be extra vigilant. If you are in any doubt, call the doctor.

Which remedy?

● If the baby is very bad-tempered, and tries to double up with the pain, but gentle pressure or massage on the abdomen from the palm of your hand seems to help, choose ☞ *Colocynthis*.

● When the baby is irritable, and tries to stretch out or bend backwards to ease the pain, choose ☞ *Dioscorea*.

● If the baby bring its knees up to its head to ease the pain, and he or she seems comforted by gentle pressure or massage, and warmth also helps, choose ☞ *Mag phos*.

CROUP

Causes and symptoms

Croup is a very harsh-sounding, tiring cough, usually associated with wheezing, that tends to affect mainly babies and small children. It tends to occur at night, in spasms or attacks. (General cough remedies are included on page 56.)

✓ Carry out the helpful measures as described for coughs (see page 56).

✓ If a child suffers a very bad attack of croup, and has great difficulty breathing, so that he or she begins to look pale or blue, get emergency medical help.

Which remedy?

● If the croup includes wheezy breathing and a harsh hollow cough that comes in tiring attacks, usually at night, there are three main remedies. First choose ☞ *Aconite*.

● If Aconite does not help croup after a few hours, choose ☞ *Spongia*.

● If Spongia is also unsuccessful for croup after a few hours, choose ☞ *Hepar sulph*.

✓ Sometimes the cough is so violent and exhausting that it can cause vomiting. Be prepared for this eventuality.

✓ Stay calm as you care for a croupy child, or you may pass on your anxiety and make matters worse.

EARACHES

Causes

Earache is usually the main symptom of an infection of the middle ear. Some children are very prone to earaches and many have several episodes. Rarely, the pain is due to an object pushed into the ear, like a bead or pea.

Symptoms

The ear pain may be accompanied by fever and some degree of hearing loss, which should improve as the condition heals. The pain may spread around the head or to the jaw and neck.

Persistent or recurrent earaches can cause hearing problems that interfere with schooling. If in doubt, ask your doctor to give the child a hearing test.

✓ Encourage the child to rest in a dimly lit, quiet place, lying on whichever side is most comfortable.

✓ A warm pad placed over the ear should help to ease the ache.

✓ If the pain persists for more than two days, or makes the child scream, or pus oozes from the ear canal, get medical advice urgently.

✓ If your child gets regular ear infections, consult a homeopath. He or she may be able to advise remedies for long-term strengthening of the body's self-defence immune system.

Which remedy?

● If the symptoms appear suddenly, especially at night or after being out in the cold, and the child is also fearful, choose ☞ *Aconite*.

● If the symptoms appear suddenly, the ear throbs and looks red, and the child develops a fever, choose ☞ *Belladonna*.

● If the pain appears gradually, and you have tried Belladonna without success, choose ☞ *Ferrum phos*.

● Should the child become extremely bad-tempered because of the pain, and he or she is only soothed by being rocked or carried, choose ☞ *Chamomilla*.

● If the first stage of inflammation is over but the ear seems to be going septic or "bad", and the child is also very irritable, with a sore throat that produces thick-yellow green mucus on coughing, choose ☞ *Hepar sulph*.

● If the pain extends down to the throat, and the child has a yellow nasal discharge which is possibly blood-streaked, and she or he is also thirsty and sweaty, with bad breath and a swollen face and neck glands, choose ☞ *Mercurius*.

● If the symptoms come and go without a pattern, and the child tries to cling to you, and feels better when cared for with sympathy, in cool surroundings, choose ☞ *Pulsatilla*.

● For any earache, insert into the ear a few warmed drops of oil prepared from *Verbascum*.

ECZEMA

Causes and symptoms

Eczema, like asthma (see page 70), has an allergic origin. The two conditions are often closely linked, especially in children. Symptoms vary from small reddish patches of dry skin, to an intensely itching, "angry" red inflammation over large areas.

✓ Try different clothing materials and washing powders, in an attempt to eliminate these as trigger factors.

✓ There are many proprietary brands of moisturizing creams that can soothe the skin.

Which remedy?

● Open sores can be safely soothed with gentle applications of a cream based on the remedy *Calendula*.

● Eczema, and other skin problems such as psoriasis or acne, should not be treated at home. There is a danger of suppressing the underlying imbalance and causing further difficulties. Consult a homeopath for advice. As with asthma, the most natural and satisfactory way to treat eczema is to strengthen your child's immune system.

✓ It is vital that anything applied to the skin is hypoallergenic.

✓ If the eczema becomes very severe or infected, consult a medical doctor.

RUBELLA (GERMAN MEASLES)

Symptoms

Rubella is usually a very mild infection, which can normally be allowed to take its course without interference. The pink skin rash may be accompanied by watery eyes and swollen glands.

Rubella is infectious for about a week after the rash appears, as well as for a few days before. It is very important that she or he avoids contact with pregnant women, because of the risk to the unborn baby. If in doubt, consult a doctor.

Which remedy?

● If the rash seems to be developing very slowly, and the child is very thirsty, wants to lie still, and is irritable, choose ☞ *Bryonia*.

● If the child's eyes are causing the most problems, being very sore and watery, choose ☞ *Euphrasia*.

● For the child with a yellow-green nasal discharge, who prefers to be cool and is not especially thirsty, but who may be slightly weepy, choose ☞ *Pulsatilla*.

● When the child has flu-like symptoms, with aching muscles and shivering, and little thirst, choose ☞ *Gelsemium*.

EMOTIONAL UPSETS

Types of problems

Most children suffer temporary behavioural or emotional difficulties at some time. These include temper tantrums, nightmares, constant crying, periods of withdrawal, and frustration showing in various ways, from screaming fits to destructiveness. Sometimes the causes of emotional upsets are obvious, such as stress at school, sibling rivalry, or frustration in learning. However other cases baffle even the experts. Remedies can help to calm the excited child and restore a sense of proportion to the situation.

✓ Always try talking and understanding first. If you can see the cause, you are halfway to the solution. Children need to know they have safe boundaries, are cared for, and are understood. Humour can also have its place.

✓ Check that your child is not sensitive to or allergic to any food additives, medications, or similar substances. These can cause behavioural problems.

✓ When you feel that you do not know how to help, consider giving one of the six constitutional remedies described on pages 32-47.

✓ For persistent problems, consult a homeopath, who will treat the child holistically.

Which remedy?

● If the child is very fearful, especially at night, and does not seem to have recovered from a previous fright, choose ☞ *Aconite*.

● For the child who lacks confidence, and who is clinging and possibly jealous of siblings, choose ☞ *Pulsatilla*.

● If the child is extremely bad-tempered and almost unapproachable, and nothing seems to please, and the problem may be connected with pain such as teething, choose ☞ *Chamomilla*.

● For the child who is shaking with fear at the thought of a forthcoming ordeal, choose ☞ *Gelsemium*.

● If the child seems very sensitive and even hysterical, choose ☞ *Ignatia*.

● For a child who is domineering and even abusive one minute, and then timid and lacking in confidence the next, choose ☞ *Lycopodium*.

● When a child will not tell you about the problem, and cries alone in his or her room, choose ☞ *Natrum muriaticum*.

● If the child is seething with anger and indignation, and cannot let go of the problem, choose ☞ *Staphysagria*.

MEASLES

Causes and symptoms

Measles is a very infectious viral disease, mainly affecting young children. It is much rarer than it used to be.

Symptoms

The characteristic early symptom is small white spots in the mouth, on the insides of the cheeks. The other main symptoms are fever, nasal discharge, and a bad cough. The rash follows, beginning on the face and spreading in blotches to the torso, but less often to the arms and legs. The eyes may hurt in bright light.

The blotches of the rash gradually merge after 5-6 days, as the fever falls. By this time the child is usually feeling better.

The remedies suggested here can help the body to fight the infection more effectively.

✓ Measles is not normally harmful in a healthy child. But inform your doctor, since rarely there can be complications.

✓ Keep the child in bed in a dimly lit, warm but well ventilated room.

✓ Give plenty of liquids until the child's temperature drops back to normal.

Which remedy?

● If the child's fever started suddenly, and he or she has a harsh barking cough, a runny nose, and red eyes, choose ☞ *Aconite*.

● When the child has a burning fever and is extremely restless, yet also drowsy and without thirst, and with puffy red eyes, choose ☞ *Apis*.

● When the fever began suddenly, and the child's pupils are widened so that she or he cannot stand the light, and the face is red and flushed, but there is no great thirst, choose ☞ *Belladonna*.

● If the rash develops slowly or stays pale, and the child has a dry painful chesty cough, a desire for long drinks of cold water, and wishes to lie still since moving is painful, choose ☞ *Bryonia*.

● If symptoms develop slowly and resemble a bad cold, with tiredness, headache, heavy eyelids, aching muscles, and shivering but no thirst, and the child feels alternately hot and cold, choose ☞ *Gelsemium*.

● If the rash is followed by a thick yellow nasal discharge and sticky eyelids, and the child has a dry cough which is worse at night, is better in a cool room, and has no great thirst, choose ☞ *Pulsatilla*.

The remedy Apis, derived from the venom of a bee's sting, is well suited to infections that cause swelling and redness.

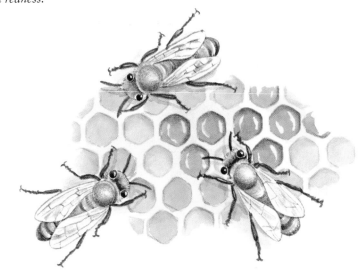

MUMPS

Causes and symptoms

Mumps is a viral disease. The salivary glands in front of the ears swell, so that the cheeks and jaw look lumpy. The fever can last up to 10 days. The child may find it painful to eat and to take sharp-tasting or sour drinks.

✓ Mumps is rarely serious, but inform your doctor, since there can be complications. In certain cases the infection and swelling can spread to the testes (testicles) of a boy, or to the ovaries of a girl. However these complications are extremely rare.

✓ Let the child rest during the feverish phase, and give plenty of drinks. If he or she has difficulty chewing, give soups.

Which remedy?

● If the symptoms appear suddenly, and the child is anxious, restless, and thirsty, choose ☞ *Aconite*.

● When the swollen glands feel tender and they look extremely puffy and red, and the child is restless and hot, and he or she wants to be kept cool but is not thirsty, choose ☞ *Apis*.

● If the illness comes on slowly, and the glands feel hard, tender, and painful, and the child is irritable, very thirsty, and wants to stay still because moving hurts, choose ☞ *Bryonia*.

● For the child with copious saliva and bad breath, and who is sweaty, thirsty, cross, and alternately hot and cold, choose ☞ *Mercurius*.

● If the child is weepy and clings on, and he or she wants to be in a cool place and is not thirsty, choose ☞ *Pulsatilla*.

● If the child is very restless, but feels better when warm, choose ☞ *Rhus tox*.

TEETHING

Causes and symptoms

Most babies and young children feel discomfort as the first set of teeth appear. A homeopathic remedy may ease the pain.

✓ Give the baby or child frequent sips of a cooling drink.

✓ The child may benefit from chewing on a clean teething ring or similar object.

Which remedy?

● If the baby is extremely bad-tempered, to the point of throwing things across the room, but he or she is helped by being carried or rocked gently, choose ☞ *Chamomilla*.

● When the baby whimpers and whines and clings on, but he or she is calmer in a cool room, choose ☞ *Pulsatilla*.

WHOOPING COUGH

Causes

Whooping cough (pertussis), a bacterial infection, affects mainly the breathing airways and lungs.

Symptoms and progression

The symptoms usually start like a cold, with a slight fever, and runny nose.

The cough develops and worsens about a week later. The "whoop" is produced when the sufferer gasps and breathes in after the coughing spasm, to bring up thick mucus trapped in the lungs. The illness can continue for weeks and be very distressing.

Whooping cough is one of the regular childhood immunizations. However some children may be advised against the immunization because of their family medical history. Homeopathic remedies can support the body's fight-back against the infection, but you should also follow your doctor's advice.

Which remedy?

In the early stages, before the typical whoop starts, you may not know the illness is whooping cough, so treat as for a cold or flu (see page 55). As the cough worsens, try a remedy suited to cough or croup (see pages 56 and 72). Then as the characteristic "whoop" begins, try one of the following remedies:

● If the cough is dry, harsh, and very painful, and it is made worse by eating and drinking (despite a marked thirst), and the child holds her or his chest while coughing because of the pain, choose ☞ *Bryonia*.

● If the child complains that the cough is caused by a ticklish feeling in the throat, and coughing spasms sometimes end in vomiting, with stringy mucus around the mouth, choose ☞ *Coccus cacti*.

● If the cough is deep and barking and seems never-ending, and it appears to come from the abdomen, and the child retches or vomits afterwards, and feels worse at night and when lying down, choose ☞ *Drosera*.

● If the child is often nauseous and vomits up mucus, and she or he has a mucus-filled rattling chest that gives a feeling of suffocation, choose ☞ *Ipecac*.

✓ Whooping cough may be especially severe in children under one year of age.

✓ It is vital to inform your doctor of the illness and follow the advice on medical care, in addition to any homeopathic remedies.

✓ Allow the child to sit up and lean forwards, which is usually the most comfortable position, during coughing spasms.

✓ Counteract the tendency to vomit when coughing by giving small meals just after a coughing bout.

Allergies

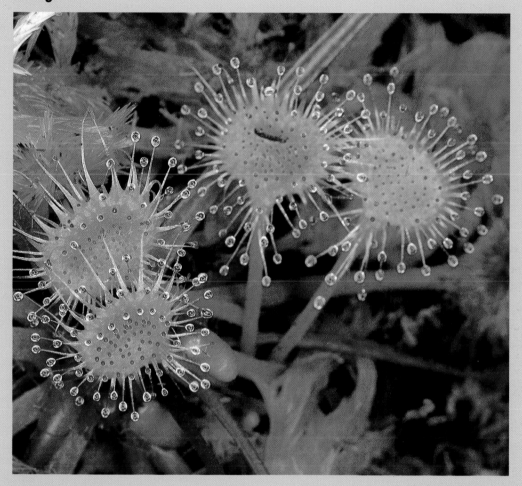

An allergy occurs when the body becomes over-sensitive to a normally harmless substance, and fights against it as though it were harmful. Allergies have become more common in recent years, probably due to a combination of environmental, dietary, and other factors. The remedy Drosera, from the sundew plant (above), can alleviate incessant coughs that may be exacerbated by allergies.

ASTHMA

Causes

Asthma is the narrowing of the small airways (bronchioles) in the lungs, as the result of an allergic reaction. The airways fill with mucus and obstruct the airflow. The primary cause is a weakened immune system, often due to a complex combination of many factors, from genetic inheritance to diet and medical drugs.

There are many possible secondary causes or triggers of asthma, from plant pollen to house dust or animal fur, dairy or wheat products, cold air, exercise, and stress. The condition is especially common among children (see page 70).

Symptoms

The key symptoms are wheezing and breathlessness. Attacks can vary from mild wheeziness to extremely frightening incidents when it seems you are fighting for every breath.

Which remedy?

The following remedies are suitable for easing mild attacks. If you become extremely breathless and the usual measures are having no effect, obtain emergency medical help.

● When attacks tend to occur at night (12am-3am), and you feel better if you sit up or walk around, and you may become tired or even exhausted after the attack, choose ☞ *Arsenicum*.

● If you feel particularly irritable or even angry during an attack, choose ☞ *Chamomilla*.

● Should tension, irritation, or outright anger seem to trigger the attack, choose ☞ *Chamomilla*.

● If you feel nauseous, your chest seems full of mucus that you cannot cough up, and you feel better in fresh air, choose ☞ *Ipecac*.

● If you are normally an affectionate and dependent person, and the attacks make you feel worse if you are in a hot stuffy room, but they are eased by cool fresh air, choose ☞ *Pulsatilla*.

● If the attacks are triggered by damp, or wet weather, or a cold, or exertion, and they tend to happen in the early hours of the morning, choose ☞ *Nat sulph*.

✓ Orthodox medical treatment usually involves anti-inflammatory drugs given by inhaler. Homeopathic remedies can be used safely with such medication.

✓ A severe asthma attack can be life-threatening. Get emergency medical help.

✓ Consult a homeopath to discuss long-term treatment aimed at strengthening the immune system to ease the problem. However this may take some time.

HAYFEVER

Causes and symptoms

Hayfever is an allergic reaction of the nose, eyes, and sometimes throat. It is usually caused by the tiny floating grains of pollen from plants, especially grasses, blossoms, and some trees. House dust, animal fur, or bird feathers may produce a similar reaction.

The main symptoms are runny, itching nose and eyes, severe sneezing, and perhaps a tickly throat. These usually come on during the particular season when the pollen is plentiful, such as midsummer for flower pollen, and last a few hours. Take the remedy at the first sign of symptoms.

The remedy Allium cepa is based on red onion – which also produces streaming eyes and a runny nose.

✓ Consider the cause of the allergy. Is it more common at a certain time of year, or near particular plants? Take steps to reduce exposure, by staying indoors.

✓ Wear dark glasses to reduce the eye irritation caused by bright light.

✓ Dry your bedding and clothes indoors, to prevent coating by pollen.

✓ Consult a homeopath to discuss long-term treatment to strengthen the immune system.

Which remedy?

● If your nose streams with a burning discharge, your eyes sting with watery tears, and you also sneeze violently, choose ☞ *Allium cepa.*

● When your nose becomes stuffed up inside, yet you still have a burning watery discharge from it and from your eyes, and you cannot stop sneezing while the attack lasts, choose ☞ *Arsenicum.*

● If your eyes are worse than your nose, and the tears burn your skin but the watery nasal discharge does not, choose ☞ *Euphrasia.*

● For constant itching in your nose, where one nostril may be blocked but the other one remains free, and the hay fever is made worse by the scents of flowers, and your eyes are sore and watering, and the sneezing is almost constant, choose ☞ *Sabadilla.*

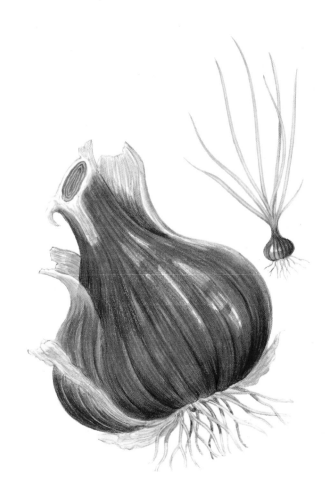

Emotional Strains and Stress

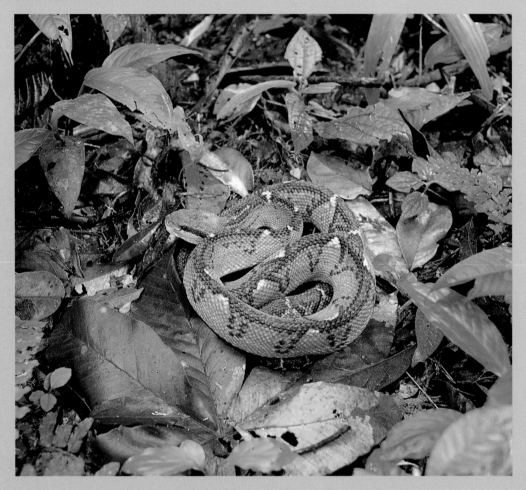

The ups and downs of modern life place many tensions and strains on our minds and our relationships with others. Homeopathic remedies and the philosophy behind them may help to ease stress and bring calm, so that we have time to step back and keep things in perspective. The remedy Lachesis, prepared from the venom of the bushmaster snake (above), is just one of the many remedies which can help with emotional problems.

ANXIETY AND PANIC

Causes and types

Worry or even panic about a future event often causes more problems than the event itself. Many people have phobias about situations such as taking exams, attending an interview, travelling in a train or plane, meeting new people, or speaking in public.

With support and sound advice from family and friends, the event usually passes and we wonder "what all the fuss was about".

When to use remedies

The remedies suggested here can help to calm and soothe, so that you are more relaxed and keep things in proportion. Use them on an acute or short-term basis – either right at the beginning of the panic or anxiety attack, or as a preventative, before you think the problem might occur.

✓ There is rarely a substitute for talking about your worries and sharing them with a caring companion.

✓ If your worries or fears are so extreme that you are hardly able to go out or cope with strangers, the problem may become long-term and deep-seated. Visit a homeopath, who will help you to locate and treat the root cause.

Which remedy?

● When you are very anxious, so that you feel you simply cannot take any more (which may even lead to diarrhoea), and you may be fearful of dark enclosed places, choose ☞ *Arg nit*.

● When you are restless, you cannot bear to be left alone, and you need constant reassurance, choose ☞ *Arsenicum*.

● If you tremble with anxiety and panic, and your muscles feel weak and refuse to obey your will, choose ☞ *Gelsemium*.

● If you are nervous and sensitive by nature, and your anxiety is brought on by twilight shadows or sudden noises, and you feel better in company, with people around, choose ☞ *Phosphorus*.

● If you feel complete terror, even to the point of being certain that you are about to die, choose ☞ *Aconite*.

● If you are overwrought, hysterical, and tearful, choose ☞ *Ignatia*.

Arsenicum album is based on a version of arsenic oxide. The power of arsenic compounds has long fascinated people, from healers to poisoning murderers.

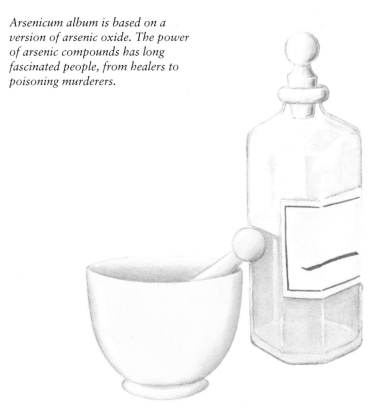

DEPRESSION

Causes and symptoms

Occasional periods of being "fed up" are normal in most of our lives. Extreme long-term sadness is more difficult to cope with. If the cause is known, try to deal with it. But sometimes there seems to be no reason.

✓ Try to talk about your feelings and problems to a sympathetic friend – someone who is perhaps not involved in the situation.

✓ Rest and a cup of tea from a caring person is probably the best remedy.

Which remedy?

● Depression usually needs outside help, from a close friend or counsellor. If it is severe or persistent, consult a medical doctor, psychiatrist, or similar professional.

● Consider some of the remedies for anxiety (see page 83) or grief (below) in milder situations.

✓ If you feel you just cannot get over the problem, it is best to see a professional.

✓ Likewise, if the depression remains for more than a few days, seek help from a trained counsellor and/or a homeopath.

GRIEF

Causes and symptoms

The sadness and loneliness we feel after losing a loved one is part of the natural grieving process, and should take its course. Homeopathy cannot remove the pain, but a remedy may ease it.

✓ If you feel that you have been "stuck" in grief for too long, consult a homeopath. He or she can help to unlock the sadness, thereby preventing future problems which might arise if it were untreated.

Which remedy?

● For the first stages of grief, when you may be weepy and very emotional, and you find yourself sighing deeply, and perhaps even becoming "hysterical", choose ☞ *Ignatia.*

● If you prefer to cry alone or you are unable to cry at all, you refuse to be consoled, and you have perhaps already tried Ignatia, choose ☞ *Natricum muriaticum.*

● If you are constantly crying, but feel better with the sympathy and consolation of others, choose ☞ *Pulsatilla.*

● If you feel emotionally "bottled up" with tears just beneath the surface, and you harbour anger or indignation about what has happened, choose ☞ *Staphysagria.*

Accidents, Emergencies, and Injuries

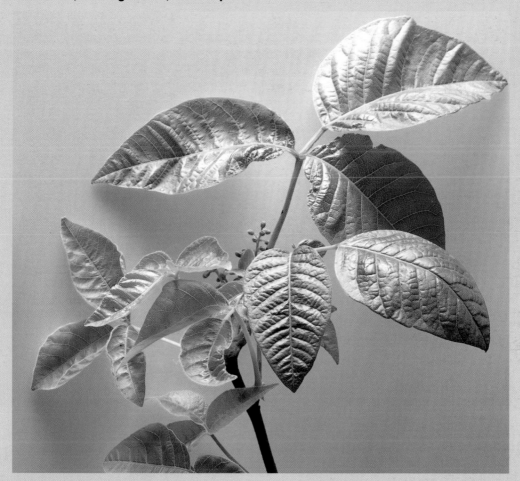

The remedy Rhus tox is prepared from the North American poison ivy plant (above). Using the homeopathic principle of "like cures like", it is an important remedy for treating sprains, strains, swollen joints, and various injuries, as well as other first aid situations. In an emergency, do not forget the basic rules of first aid: save life, summon help, make the casualty safe and comfortable, and then begin treatment.

BITES AND STINGS

Causes and symptoms

Minor bites and stings cause few problems if you are otherwise healthy. Use one of these remedies to ease the pain or if you feel you are healing too slowly.

✓ Always clean the wound. Use tweezers to remove any sting.

✓ Rub Calendula or Hypercal cream, or a diluted (1 in 10) tincture of these remedies, into the wound with a cotton pad. This acts as an antiseptic.

Which remedy?

● If the injury swells, burns, and stings, and also looks red and "angry", choose ☞ *Apis*.

● When there is bruising and soreness in addition to the bite or sting itself, choose ☞ *Arnica*.

● If burning pain is the worst symptom, choose ☞ *Cantharis*.

● If you suspect that the animal responsible may be very poisonous, or if there is a risk of an allergic reaction, get medical help as quickly as possible.

BOILS

Causes and symptoms

A boil is an infected, swollen, reddened area of skin around a hair follicle (the pit from which the hair grows). Boils can be very painful while they develop, until they come to a head and burst to discharge the pus.

✓ Bathe the boil in hot salted water to encourage it to "gather" and discharge.

✓ If you are still in pain or the boil has not come to a head after a few days, ask your homeopath or doctor for help.

Which remedy?

● If the boil is hot and burning, yet hot compresses ease the pain, choose ☞ *Arsenicum*.

● When the boil has come up quickly, and looks red and "angry", and throbs violently, choose ☞ *Belladonna*.

● If the pains are very sharp and penetrating, and get worse when you are cold, and the boil seems to be full of oozing yellow-green pus, choose ☞ *Hepar sulph*.

● For a boil that appears to have gone septic or "bad", and you feel that there is some foreign body buried inside it which will not come out, choose ☞ *Silica*.

● If the boil developed rapidly after a slow start, and now feels hard, burning, and very painful, and it looks blue-tinged in colour, choose ☞ *Tarentula cubensis*.

BRUISES

Causes and symptoms

The black-and-blue appearance of a bruise is caused by blood vessels rupturing under the unbroken skin, following heavy pressure. As the blood breaks down and is reabsorbed, the bruise becomes paler and then red or yellow.

✓ Always ensure any wounds are cleaned first.

✓ If possible, rest the bruised part in a sling or splint to encourage healing.

Which remedy?

● For bruises and other injuries where the skin is unbroken, choose ☞ *Arnica*. Apply it directly as a cream, or take it by mouth in the usual pill form. For severe bruising, use both the cream and pill.

● If the bruise is on a sensitive area such as the fingertip, lip, nose, or coccyx (base of the spine), and the pain shoots along the tracks of the nerves, choose ☞ *Hypericum* or *Hypercal*. Apply directly to the site as a cream or diluted tincture (one part of tincture in ten parts of water).

● If you feel that your bones have been deeply bruised, for example, after a knock or kick on the shin, choose ☞ *Ruta*.

BURNS

Causes and symptoms

These remedies are for minor burns, including sunburn and scalding from hot liquids.

Minor burns are painful but limited in area and depth, so they give no cause for alarm.

✓ As a general guide, any burned area larger that the victim's hand should be seen by a doctor.

✓ So should any burn, no matter what size, that has penetrated the skin to expose the flesh beneath.

✓ Drink plenty of fluids, to prevent dehydration from loss of body fluids.

Which remedy?

● If the victim is shocked, choose ☞ *Arnica* as a first remedy (see page 92).

● When the burn is fairly minor, and is reddened but not blistering, apply *Urtica* or *Calendula* or *Hypercal*. Rub it gently onto the area with a cotton wool swab, either as a cream or a diluted tincture (one part of tincture in ten parts of water).

● If the burn begins to blister, choose ☞ *Cantharis* or *Causticum*, and take as a pill every hour.

● For a serious burn, when you are seeking medical help, choose ☞ *Cantharis* or *Causticum*. Take as a pill every 15 minutes while waiting for attention.

CUTS AND SORES

Causes and symptoms

These remedies should help when the skin is broken by a sharp object, or when it is red and sore. Observe the usual first aid guidelines, such as cleaning the wound of dirt and foreign objects.

✓ Cover deep or wide cuts with a sticking plaster or bandage, and avoid immersion in water.

✓ If a wound is large or gaping, or does not stop bleeding after 20-30 minutes, obtain urgent medical help.

Which remedy?

● If the skin is not broken, choose ☞ *Arnica* (see page 87).

● For small cuts or sores (except those described below), apply a cream or diluted tincture (one part of tincture in ten parts of water) of *Calendula*. Rub it gently into the site with a cotton wool swab.

● If the wound is on a sensitive area such as a fingertip or lip, and the pain shoots along a nearby nerve, choose ☞ *Hypericum* or *Hypercal*. Apply as a cream or diluted tincture (one part of tincture to ten parts of water).

● If you suffer a puncture wound, and the injury feels cold to the touch, and is relieved by cold compresses, choose ☞ *Ledum*. Either take it as a pill, or apply it as a diluted tincture (one part of tincture in ten parts of water).

EYE INJURIES AND STRAIN

Causes and symptoms

Eyes are very delicate. They are sensitive to physical knocks and injury, and they tire easily from the strain of watching a TV screen or reading in poor light.

✓ Avoid strain. Rest eyes regularly.

✓ Do not spend more than an hour or two in front of a TV or computer screen without a break.

✓ For an eye injury, wash your hands first and then bathe the eye in sterile (boiled and cooled) water.

✓ Never take chances with eyes. Seek medical advice sooner, not later.

Which remedy?

● For an eye injury accompanied by bruising, choose ☞ *Arnica* as a first remedy.

● If the eye becomes cold and bloodshot after a blow, choose ☞ *Ledum*. Take it as a pill or apply it as a diluted tincture (a few drops of tincture in a small glass of water) to the eye.

● If you suffer from general eye strain and your eyes water and burn, choose ☞ *Euphrasia*. Apply it as a diluted tincture (a few drops of tincture in a small glass of water) to the eye.

● If your eyes become sore and your vision seems dim after too much close work, choose ☞ *Ruta*.

EYE INFLAMMATION

Causes and symptoms

Blepharitis is redness, soreness, and swelling of the eyelid. Conjunctivitis is inflammation of the conjunctiva – the delicate, moist membrane that covers the front of the eye. These problems can affect one or both eyes.

✓ To soothe eyes, see below.

✓ Seek medical advice if there are visual problems, or if inflammation does not start to clear after two days.

Which remedy?

● If your eye feels hot and dry, and it seems like a piece of grit has got into it, and the eye looks red and inflamed, perhaps as a result of being in a cold wind or draught, choose ☞ *Aconite*.

● When the eyeball seems burning, and it appears red, swollen, and filled with fluid, but feels better with a cold compress, choose ☞ *Apis*.

● If your eye is very sensitive to light, with a dilated pupil, and it also feels burning and dry, and looks bloodshot, choose ☞ *Belladonna*.

● For the eye that burns and waters, and has a sticky eyelid, choose ☞ *Euphrasia*. Place a few drops of tincture in a small glass of water and bathe the eye with this.

● If the eye is swollen and sore, with a watery yellow discharge and perhaps sticky lids as well, choose ☞ *Pulsatilla*.

STYES

Causes and symptoms

A stye is a small boil on the eyelid, affecting the follicle of an eyelash hair. In severe cases the eyelid may swell and close. Consider these remedies and those for eye inflammation (above) and boils (see page 86).

✓ To soothe eyes, bathe them in sterile (boiled and cooled) water or apply a compress of a clean pad soaked in sterile cold water.

✓ Seek medical advice if there are visual problems, or if inflammation does not start to clear after two days.

Which remedy?

● When styes keep recurring, and they discharge mainly yellow pus, choose ☞ *Pulsatilla*.

● For a stye that appears after a period of emotional stress, which you have bottled up or suppressed, choose ☞ *Staphysagria*.

● For a stye near the inner canthus – where the eyelids meet the nose – and which itches, choose ☞ *Lycopodium*.

● For a painful stye, where the pain seems hot and burning, choose ☞ *Sulphur*.

FAINTING AND COLLAPSE

Causes and symptoms

Faintness or collapse have many causes, including emotional shock, pain, fright, tiredness, or hunger. Very occasionally, it is due to a more serious illness.

The symptoms include feeling cold, clammy, and dizzy, and turning pale. In a full faint or collapse, the person loses consciousness and falls to the floor. This is a self-protection mechanism, to restore adequate blood flow to the brain.

Usually the unconsciousness is brief. Carry out first aid measures, in conjunction with the remedies advised here. For medical shock, see page 92.

✓ Make sure the person is lying down or leaning back, and keep warm and as comfortable as possible. Try to get the head lower than the legs, to restore blood flow to the brain. Otherwise, do not move the person until he or she feels ready.

✓ Try to keep curious people away and ensure some privacy. As the person recovers, offer sips of water.

✓ If he or she remains unconscious, moisten the lips with Rescue remedy every few minutes.

✓ If the faintness has not passed after 10-15 minutes, get emergency medical help.

✓ If this is the first faint that the person has had, consult a doctor.

Which remedy?

● Always give the Bach Flower remedy known as the *Rescue remedy* (see page 137). In addition:

● When the person collapses from intense fright, and perhaps cannot get over the fright afterwards, choose ☞ *Aconite.*

● If there is shock from an accident or from great physical pain, choose ☞ *Arnica.*

● If the person feels cold, and is slow in coming round, and seems exhausted afterwards, choose ☞ *Carbo veg.*

● For fainting linked to loss of fluids, such as vomiting, diarrhoea, or loss of blood, choose ☞ *China.*

● If the fainting is caused by emotional shock, such as hearing bad news, choose ☞ *Ignatia.*

● When the fainting may be caused by stuffy, airless surroundings, choose ☞ *Pulsatilla.*

The dried bark of the Peruvian cinchona or quinine tree yields the remedy China.

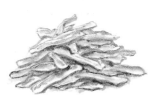

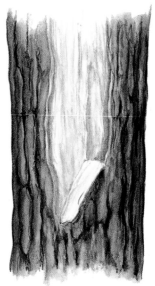

FRACTURES

Causes and symptoms

A fractured (broken) bone needs hospital treatment, but remedies can aid healing. The bones are usually put back into their natural positions for healing. The body part may be protected by a casing or plaster for up to six weeks.

✓ If you suspect a fracture, from extreme pain or a misshapen body part, summon expert first aid. Moving the part could make the injury worse.

Which remedy?

● For the bruising and shock, as in any accident, choose ☞ *Arnica*.

● If Arnica does not seem to help the bruising, choose ☞ *Ruta*.

● When the pain from the broken bone is agonizing from the slightest movement, so that you feel you must keep perfectly still, choose ☞ *Bryonia*.

● After the broken parts of the bone have been re-positioned ("reduced" or "set"), choose ☞ *Symphytum*. Take this in pill form daily for a month to help the bone parts knit together. (The remedy comes from the herb comfrey, also called boneset.)

● When the initial healing is completed after about one month, choose ☞ *Calc phos*. Take this in pill form daily until you feel fully recovered.

NOSEBLEEDS

Causes and symptoms

Nosebleeds can be caused by an injury or violent sneeze, but some occur for no obvious reason. They usually stop on their own, or after simple first aid (see below). One of these remedies may help to promote healing.

✓ Help to staunch the bleeding by applying pressure to the upper nose. This is usually done by pinching the nose on the soft part just below the bony bridge, for 10-15 minutes.

✓ A cold compress on the nose may also help to stop the bleeding.

Which remedy?

● If the bleeding is due to a knock on the nose or some other physical injury, choose ☞ *Arnica*.

● When the bleeding starts without an obvious cause, choose ☞ *Phosphorus*.

● If Phosphorus does not seem to help, choose ☞ *Lachesis*.

✓ Lean forwards, with the face looking slightly down, while carrying out first aid. Allow the blood to drain, rather than sniffing it inwards.

✓ Do not blow the nose for six or eight hours, or you may dislodge the blood clot and restart the bleeding.

SHOCK

Causes

The medical condition of shock is is due a sudden fall in the amount of blood circulating through parts of the body, especially the brain and other vital organs. This may result from bleeding, when various tissues and organs are starved of the vital, life-giving oxygen carried by the blood.

Shock can result from a serious physical injury, although the damage may be internal and so not obvious. It may also be due to emotional reasons.

Symptoms

The symptoms include a weak pulse, shallow breathing, cold pale skin, anxiety, feeling faint, confusion, and perhaps unconsciousness.

✓ Get medical help immediately if the shock follows a bad accident or seems inexplicable.

✓ Keep the person warm and loosen any tight clothing.

✓ Do not move the person if there is a serious injury or if he or she is unconscious.

✓ But do ensure the head is in a low position compared to the body and limbs, to maintain blood flow to the head and brain.

Which remedy?

● Give the **Rescue remedy** immediately. If the person is unconscious, a few drops on the lips will be adequate.

● Always give **Arnica** as well. It is the foremost remedy for shock, as well as for bruising and similar physical injury.

● If the person is conscious and very frightened, choose ☞ **Aconite**.

● If the shock may have an emotional reason, choose ☞ **Ignatia**.

● Should the shock be due to sudden fluid loss, choose ☞ **China**.

● In an emergency, give the remedies every few minutes.

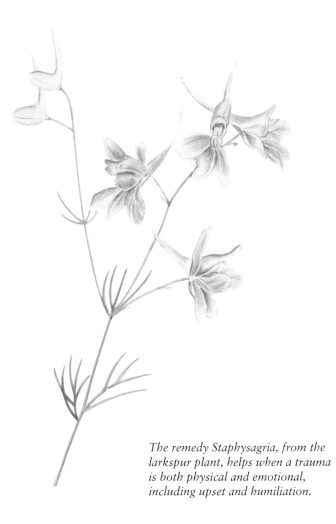

The remedy Staphysagria, from the larkspur plant, helps when a trauma is both physical and emotional, including upset and humiliation.

SPRAINS AND STRAINS

Causes and symptoms

These joint problems are due to twisting, wrenching, or over-use. A sprain is damaged tendons or ligaments. A strain happens when the connecting tissues around a joint are over-stretched.

✓ Obtain urgent medical help if the problem affects a major joint or if the person is in great pain.

✓ Cool the joint with cold compresses and then support it with a bandage, but not tied too tightly.

Which remedy?

● As a general rule, choose ☞ *Arnica*. Apply it as a cream or diluted tincture (one part of tincture in ten parts of water) to any bruised or painful area.

● If the pain worsens on the slightest movement, so that you have to support or hold the injured part tightly, choose ☞ *Bryonia*.

● When the injured part looks purple and puffy, and it feels cold, yet cold compresses help to ease the pain, choose ☞ *Ledum*.

● If the pain is worse immediately after the injury, but then it begins to ease as you start to move and bend the joint, and the pain or discomfort is helped by warmth, gentle massage, and a supporting bandage, choose ☞ *Rhus tox*.

● If the bones inside and near the joint feel bruised, choose ☞ *Ruta*.

AFTER SURGERY AND DENTAL TREATMENT

Causes and symptoms

Many people become extremely worried before they visit a doctor, dentist, or hospital for minor surgical procedures. The worry can also continue afterwards and interfere with healing.

Remedies that can help to calm you before you attend are included under Anxiety and Panic (see page 83). If you feel that you are still suffering physical or emotional trauma after the treatment, then try one of the remedies described here.

Which remedy?

● For any general shock or bruising, choose ☞ *Arnica*.

● For open cuts and wounds, choose ☞ *Calendula*. Apply it as a cream or diluted tincture (one part of tincture to ten parts of water), rubbing it gently into the affected area.

● When the nerve endings are injured, which causes shooting pains along the nearby nerves, choose ☞ *Hypericum*.

● If there is excessive bleeding, especially after a tooth extraction, choose ☞ *Phosphorus*.

● When you feel very vague, detached, and "spacey" as a result of an anaesthetic, choose ☞ *Phosphorus*.

● If you feel upset and humiliated because of the insensitivity shown by the dentist or surgeon (even though it was unintentional), and this seems to be slowing the healing process, choose ☞ *Staphysagria*.

TOOTHACHES

Causes

Toothache can be caused by various conditions, such as dental decay (caries), or gum inflammation (gingivitis), or possibly infection. Another cause is an infected area of tissue and bone called an abscess, that may be visible at the surface of the gum, or down inside the jawbone and so hidden.

Symptoms

Toothache can vary from a mild discomfort to an intense pain that blocks out almost all other awareness. It may be continuous, or come in throbbing spasms. As it progresses and spreads, it can be difficult to identify the exact tooth involved.

The remedies advised here will not cure the underlying cause, but they may ease the pain until you can visit the dentist.

Which remedy?

● If the abscess comes up very quickly (in a few hours), and the infected area looks red, hot, and swollen, and the tooth throbs painfully, choose ☞ *Belladonna*.

● When the pain feels very sharp, jagged, and "splintery", and the affected area looks obviously infected and even septic with swelling and pus, and it is very sensitive to touch and cold air, and also you generally feel very cross, choose ☞ *Hepar sulph*.

● For gums that feel very sore and keep bleeding, with pus present at the infection site, and when your breath is bad, and you are producing copious saliva, choose ☞ *Mercurius*.

● If the abscess does not seem to be "gathering" and coming to a head, or if it has passed its worst but it is being slow to heal, and especially if your teeth are generally not in a very healthy condition, choose ☞ *Silica*.

● When the pain makes you very bad-tempered, and you cannot bear people near you, choose ☞ *Chamomilla*.

● If you feel better, and the pain is relieved by sympathy from others and fresh cool air, choose ☞ *Pulsatilla*.

✓ There is no real substitute for seeing the dentist, who can deal with the underlying cause.

✓ The swelling and pressure of an abscess may be helped by applying hot compresses to the affected site.

✓ Wash out your mouth every hour or so with warm salt water, to soothe any inflammation.

✓ Any dental problem is less likely if you take good care of your teeth and gums.

✓ Important guidelines for good dental care are to brush your teeth regularly, cut down on sweet and sugary foods and drinks, and also floss your teeth. Your dentist or hygienist can show you how and give further advice.

TRAVEL SICKNESS

Causes and symptoms

Car, boat, and air sickness, and nausea after a violent fairground ride, have the same basic cause. The ear's balance mechanism uses fluid moving in tiny tubes. It is upset as the fluid whirls around, and sends confused information to the brain. This does not match information from the eyes about what you see, or the strange body posture to remain balanced. The conflicting and unfamiliar activity in the brain brings on nausea (feeling sick), dizziness, and actual vomiting. There may also be abdominal pains, and signs of anxiety such as panting, sweating, and fast pulse.

✓ Avoid eating large meals before you travel. In particular, do not eat rich and heavy foods.

✓ If you feel thirsty, drink sips of plain water rather than tea, coffee, or alcohol.

✓ Try to expose yourself to fresh air or air-conditioning, especially on your face. If you are on a boat, go up on deck. In a plane or bus, adjust the air vent to give a cooling light breeze.

✓ In a boat, sit where you can see the water and horizon through a window.

✓ Avoid reading or doing other activities that require mental concentration and detailed use of the eyes.

Which remedy?

The two chief remedies for travel or motion sickness are **Cocculus** and **Tabacum**. Even if your symptom picture does not fit very closely, it is worth trying one or the other.

● If you have all the general symptoms of travel or motion sickness, and you just want to lie down, and even the thought of food makes you nauseous, choose ☞ **Cocculus**.

● If you are sweating, and you look very pale, and you feel better in cool fresh air, choose ☞ **Tabacum**.

● If you cannot get over the shock of the problem, even some time later, choose ☞ **Arnica**.

The common tobacco plant is used to prepare the remedy Tabacum, an important treatment for travel sickness.

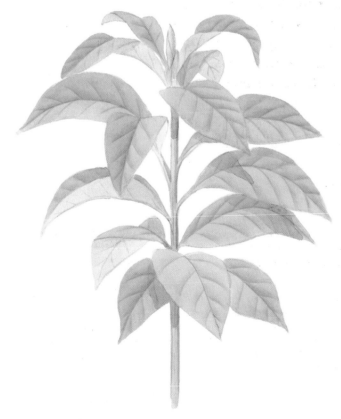

Chapter Four

A Guide to Remedies

This chapter contains descriptions and symptom pictures or patterns for about 60 of the most useful and most commonly used homeopathic remedies. It is a form of Materia Medica (see page 12), although it has been shortened and made easier to use. The Materia Medicas used by experienced homeopaths cover hundreds of remedies and some of them run for thousands of pages!

Remedies are usually available in pill or tablet form, from pharmacists, health stores, mail order organizations, and other suppliers, as described at the end of the book. Sometimes they can be bought in powder or liquid form. The first aid remedies such as Arnica or Calendula can also be supplied as creams or tinctures.

Making remedies

Each remedy is diluted and succussed many times, in accordance with homeopathic principles. The final dilution is incorporated into the pill made of a simple, inert carrier substance, usually sucrose-lactose, which makes up the main bulk of the pill. This has been succussed with the remedy at the relevant potency, to absorb it.

A few people make their own remedies from original ingredients. However it is a long and complex process. The dilution and the succussion require skilled training if they are to be effective. It may also be very difficult to track down the correct ingredients. The commercially available pills are ideal for both home and professional use. They are inexpensive, readily available, and easy to use.

> "*Aude sapere* – Have the courage to think for yourself."
>
> Motto of Samuel Hahnemann, founder of modern homeopathy (see page 11). It encourages people to take on more responsibility for their own health and treatment.

The herb rue is the source of the homeopathic remedy Ruta. The whole, fresh plant is used. It must be unexposed to chemical sprays or fertilizers.

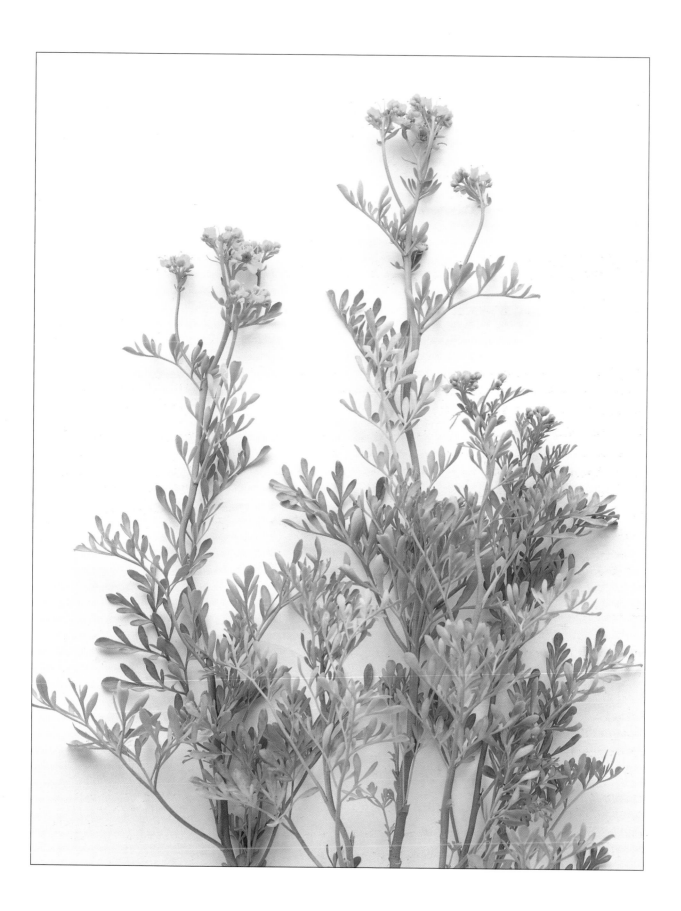

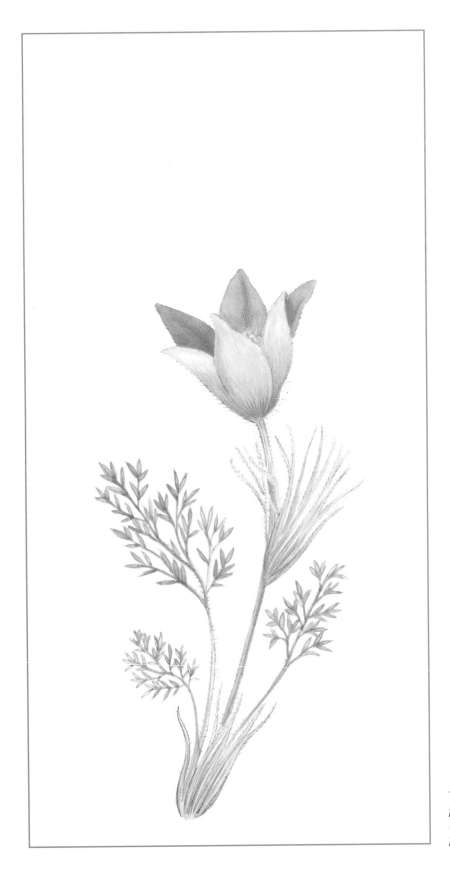

The remedy Pulsatilla is prepared from the whole fresh pasque flower (wind flower) plant, when it is in flower.

Index of Remedies

Aconite 100

Aesculus 100

Allium cepa 101

Antimonium tartaricum
(Ant tart) 101

Apis 102

Argentum nitricum
(Arg nit) 102

Arnica 103

Arsenicum album 103

Belladonna 104

Bryonia 104

Calcarea carbonica
(Calc carb) 106

Calcarea phosphorica
(Calc phos) 106

Calendula 107

Cantharis 107

Carbo vegetabilis
(Carbo veg) 109

Causticum 109

Chamomilla 110

China 110

Cocculus 111

Coccus cacti 111

Colocynthis 111

Dioscorea 113

Drosera 112

Eupatorium 113

Euphrasia 113

Ferrum phosphoricum
(Ferrum phos) 114

Gelsemium 114

Hamamelis 115

Hepar sulph
(Hepar sulphuris calcareum) 115

Hypericum 116

Ignatia 116

Ipecac (Ipecacuanha) 119

Lachesis 119

Ledum 120

Lycopodium 120

Magnesia phosphorica
(Mag phos) 121

Mercurius 121

Natrum muriaticum
(Nat mur) 122

Natrum sulphuricum
(Nat sulph) 122

Nux vomica 124

Phosphorus 124

Phytolacca 125

Podophyllum 125

Pulsatilla 126

Rhus tox 126

Rumex 128

Ruta 128

Sabadilla 129

Sarsaparilla 129

Sepia 130

Silica 130

Spongia 131

Staphysagria 131

Sulphur 133

Symphytum 133

Tabacum 135

Tarentula cubensis 135

Urtica 136

Veratrum album 136

Verbascum 137

Rescue remedy 137

ACONITE

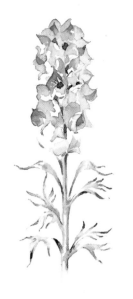

Problems helped by Aconite

Fevers, sore throats, coughs, colds, influenza, croup, earaches, and sore eyes, and also emotional states such as anxiety, fright, and shock.

Origin and actions

The remedy is derived from monkshood, a plant whose beautiful but poisonous flowers are shaped like a monk's head cowl. Aconite is best used in the first stages of an illness, especially when fear and anxiety are present.

Typical symptoms

* Symptoms appear suddenly, without warning, and they may be caused by exposure to cold winds or draughts, or by a severe fright.
* Marked restlessness.
* Extreme anxiety or fear.
* High fever with a burning skin.
* "Hot" headaches, as if there is a tight band around the head.
* Extreme sweating and a burning thirst.
* A hoarse, dry, painful cough.
* Bright light, noise, stress, and cold worsen the symptoms.
* Rest and quiet relieve the symptoms.

AESCULUS

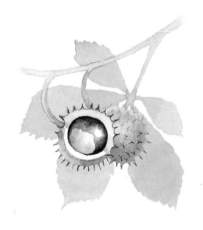

Problems helped by Aesculus

Chiefly haemorrhoids (piles) and other problems involving swollen, engorged veins.

Origin and actions

The remedy comes from the horse chestnut tree, being prepared from the ripe nuts. It acts specifically on the veins of the lower bowel, rectum, and anus. Aesculus can be used either as a cream applied directly to the swollen veins, or taken by mouth in the usual homeopathic pill form.

Typical symptoms

* The haemorrhoids are purple and painful, and feel hot and burning.
* Sharp pains shoot from the anal region up the back.
* Walking or standing still worsens the symptoms.
* Sitting comfortably in the cool, open air relieves the symptoms.
* The haemorrhoids may improve in summer and worsen in winter.

ALLIUM CEPA

Problems helped by Allium cepa

Ailments affecting the delicate membranes covering the eyes and lining the nasal passages, such as hayfever, colds, and ticklish coughs.

Origin and actions

Allium cepa, otherwise known as the red onion, acts on the mucous membranes of the eyes, nose, throat, and larynx (voice-box). It can therefore help to soothe allergies, inflammations, and infections affecting these parts.

Typical symptoms

* Sneezing, which may be violent, and occur repeatedly and frequently.
* An acrid burning discharge from the nose.
* Eyes that are runny and streaming.
* Although the eyes themselves feel burning, the tears are watery and bland.
* Being in cool, open air relieves the symptoms.

ANTIMONIUM TARTARICUM (Ant tart)

Problems helped by Antimonium tartaricum

Chickenpox, and lung problems involving thick mucus and difficult breathing.

Origin and actions

Antimonium tartaricum is prepared from the chemical tartar emetic. It affects the mucous membranes of the lungs, and helps a weak person to cough up the trapped mucus (phlegm). It also aids formation of the spots in chickenpox, which is important to ensure the disease progresses.

Typical symptoms

* Gurgling or wheezing sounds that indicate accumulated mucus in the lungs, which cannot be coughed up easily.
* Shortness of breath, which can even seem suffocating.
* A loose, rattling cough, often from deep in the chest.
* Weakness and drowsiness.
* Sweating, which may be copious, cold, and clammy.
* Chickenpox spots, when the spots will not "gather" and come to a head.

APIS

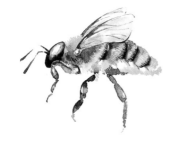

Problems helped by Apis

Various types of swelling and inflammation, such as animal bites and stings, also measles and mumps, sore throats, sore red eyes, and fevers.

Origin and actions

The remedy comes from the honey bee, and the symptom pattern mimics the bee's sting. Apis is an important quick-acting remedy where there is inflammation, and especially oedema – swelling with excessive fluid in the body tissues.

Typical symptoms

* Swelling with oedema, which makes the affected parts look shiny, red, and puffy.
* The swollen parts feel "soggy" and waterlogged.
* Burning and stinging pains.
* A fever that develops rapidly, but tends to be without thirst.
* Drowsiness but also insomnia (problems in sleeping).
* Extreme restlessness and fidgeting.
* An irritable nature, and perhaps signs of jealousy.
* Cool air and cold compresses relieve the symptoms.

ARGENTUM NITRICUM (Arg nit)

Problems helped by Argentum nitricum

Emotional states such as nervousness, anxiety, and panic attacks.

Origin and actions

Argentum nitricum is produced from a crystalline chemical, silver nitrate (also used in the preparation of photographic films). It is a major remedy for anxiety states involving anticipation, especially worry about a forthcoming event or ordeal.

Typical symptoms

* Nervousness and lack of confidence.
* Anxiety about future events that are "ordeals", such as taking a test or examination, appearing or speaking in public, travelling by plane, and so on.
* Panic that can lead to diarrhoea and bloating.
* Fright that may be so intense that it almost paralyses, as though "frozen by fear".
* Feelings of being alone and abandoned.
* Worry accompanied by hurry, feeling both anxious and rushed.

Problems helped by Arnica

Bruises and similar injuries where the skin is unbroken, and mental and physical shock.

Origin and actions

Arnica is prepared from the daisy-like herb of the same name, also known as fall herb, that usually grows in mountainous areas. It is the most important of the homeopathic injury remedies, and acts on the soft tissues, including the muscles and blood vessels. It can be applied as a cream or taken in pill form.

Typical symptoms

* Any type of bruising or similar injury caused by crushing, squeezing, or wrenching. (Arnica should be applied as the cream or ointment only if the skin is not broken. If the skin is broken, by a cut or graze, use Calendula cream.)
* Muscle strains which feel sore and bruised, such as after a fall or as a result of a sport injury.
* Shock after an accident or following collapse, in addition to the appropriate first aid treatment.

ARNICA

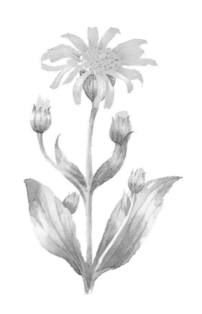

Problems helped by Arsenicum

Colds and influenza, hayfever, asthma, food poisoning and digestive upsets, and worry and anxiety.

Origin and actions

This remedy is prepared from the infamously poisonous substance arsenic (arsenious oxide). It is important for both short-term acute and long-term chronic ailments. It acts especially well on the respiratory system, and on the whole digestive tract including the stomach and intestines.

Typical symptoms

* Digestive symptoms such as vomiting, diarrhoea, and stomach cramps.
* Head colds with a thin, watery, runny nasal discharge.
* Asthmatic, wheezy breathing.
* Anxiety which responds to the comfort and support of others.
* Feeling chilly, weak, restless, and thirsty for sips of cold water.
* The symptoms seem out of proportion and too extreme for the severity of the disease.
* The symptoms worsen after midnight.
* Warmth relieves the symptoms.

ARSENICUM ALBUM

BELLADONNA

Problems helped by Belladonna

Colds, influenza, sore throats, toothaches, earaches, boils and similar inflammations, fevers, and also chickenpox, measles, and mumps.

Origin and actions

Belladonna is made from the well-know deadly nightshade, a tall plant with large, glossy, black, poisonous berries. It is a major short-term or acute remedy for all kinds of fevers and feverish illnesses, especially in the first stages.

Typical symptoms

* The symptoms appear suddenly and are already intense.
* A fever and burning, dry skin, but without a marked thirst.
* The face or other affected part is usually bright red.
* Restlessness, confusion, even delirium in severe cases.
* The eye pupils may be widened or dilated, giving a staring "wide-eyed" look.
* Any pains are felt as throbbing, especially in the head area.
* Bright light, touch, pressure, and draughts worsen the symptoms.

BRYONIA

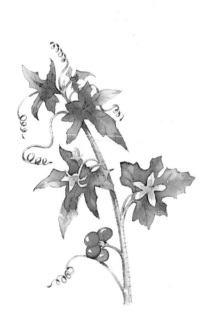

Problems helped by Bryonia

Coughs, colds, influenza, and bronchitis, also stomach upsets, headaches, mumps, and injuries such as joint sprains and minor dislocations.

Origin and actions

White bryony is a common climbing plant found throughout Europe, and its roots yield this remedy. It can help many and varied problems, but for the maximum effect, it is important that the symptom picture fits very closely.

Typical symptoms

* The symptoms and underlying ailment develop slowly.
* The affected parts – mouth, nose, lungs, joints – feel dry and unlubricated.
* Any cough is dry and painful, and eased by holding the chest.
* Extreme thirst.
* Feelings of irritability and wanting to be left alone.
* The pains are sharp and penetrating, like a "stitch".
* The slightest motion worsens the symptoms.
* Firm pressure on the affected area relieves the symptoms.

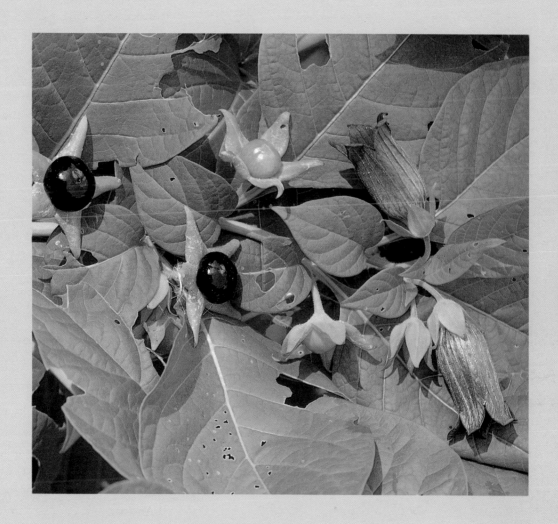

Belladonna is made from deadly nightshade, with its attractive but famously poisonous berries. During the Renaissance period, Italian ladies of fashion put the diluted juice into their eyes, to enlarge their pupils and make them look more attractive. The name Belladonna *means "beautiful lady".*

CALCAREA CARBONICA
(Calc carb)

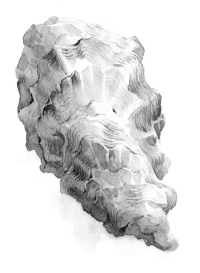

Problems helped by Calcarea carbonica

A remedy for many illnesses, provided the symptoms fit.

Origin and actions

Calcarea carbonica is made from a type of lime, prepared from the middle layer of oyster shells. It is mainly a long-term constitutional remedy, especially for children (see page 36). Its use is generally best left to a homeopathic practitioner, unless the symptom picture corresponds very closely to the descriptions.

Typical symptoms

The main symptoms and personality features are described in the constitutional profile for the Calc carb type (see page 36). Briefly these are:
* Tendencies to constipation, coughs, colds, sore throats, fevers, and ankle strains.
* A steady and methodical approach to life, its problems and events.
* A dislike of being rushed, which may show as stubbornness.
* A self-contained and independent personality, which may sometimes seem serious.

CALCAREA PHOSPHORICA
(Calc phos)

Problems helped by Calcarea phosphorica

Growing pains and aching bones in children, and healing broken bones.

Origin and actions

Calcarea phosphorica is prepared from the mineral calcium phosphate, which contains both calcium and phosphorus – two of the main constituent elements of bone. This remedy has an important part to play in bone repair and nutrition, especially in younger life.

Typical symptoms

* Bone breaks or fractures, after they have been repositioned and set, and after the remedy Symphytum (see page 133) has been used to help knit the bones back together.
* Aching bones and general growing pains in children, especially those who are tall and thin, and who are prone to headaches and swollen glands.

Problems helped by Calendula

Open wounds, cuts, sores, burns, and similar injuries.

Origin and actions

Calendula is derived from the leaves and flowers of the marigold, a familiar herb or pot-plant with deep orange petals. It is the most important first aid remedy for open wounds. Calendula not only speeds healing, it also prevents the wound from becoming infected and turning septic.

Typical symptoms

For small injuries, apply Calendula to the affected part as a cream or diluted tincture (one part of tincture to ten parts of water). For more serious wounds, it can be taken by mouth in pill form, in addition to applying the cream/tincture, and carrying out the appropriate first aid measures.
* Any type of cut or sore where the skin is broken. (For bruising and closed wounds where the skin is not broken, the main remedy is Arnica.)
* Mild burns.
* Mild stings.

CALENDULA

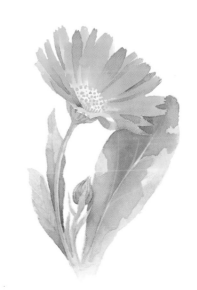

Problems helped by Cantharis

Burns and scalds of many different kinds, and the bladder inflammation of cystitis.

Origin and actions

Cantharis is prepared from an insect – the brilliant-green beetle known as the Spanish fly. It is an important first aid remedy for minor burns, and for other pains that feel burning and fiery. It also has a healing effect on the bladder, urethra, and other parts of the urinary tract, where burning pain is the key symptom.

Typical symptoms

* Small burns and scalds, especially where blistering and inflammation occur.
* Sunburn.
* Insect bites which feel hot and burning.
* Cystitis, particularly where the pain is burning or scalding.
* Other ailments where a hot or burning pain is the predominant symptom, and when the symptoms come on suddenly.

CANTHARIS

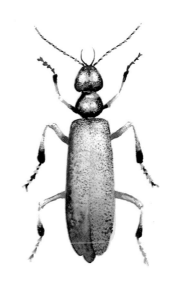

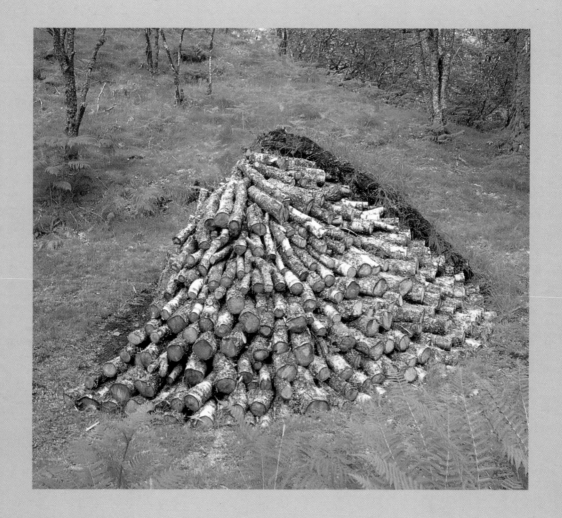

Carbo vegetabilis is based on charcoal, which itself comes in many forms. It is usually made by partially burning wood or a similar carbon-rich substance in a very slow way, with limited supplies of oxygen. Charcoal is used to absorb unwanted materials and odours, in various chemical processes, and in air filters and even fish-tank filters.

CARBO VEGETABILIS (Carbo veg)

Problems helped by Carbo vegetabilis

Fainting and collapse.

Origin and actions

Carbo vegetabilis is prepared from charcoal, which in turn is usually made by part-burning certain types of wood. This remedy is normally prescribed by a homeopath, rather than self-prescribed at home. However it can be very useful in cases of fainting, since it helps to increase the oxygen content of the circulating blood.

Typical symptoms

* Feeling faint and actual fainting or collapse (in conjunction with appropriate first aid measures).
* Associated symptoms such as dizziness, light-headedness, and general weakness.
* Coldness.
* Paleness.
* A tendency to flatulence (digestive gas or wind).
* Fresh air relieves the symptoms.

CAUSTICUM

Problems helped by Causticum

Burns and burning pains such as cystitis, also coughs.

Origin and actions

Causticum is prepared from slaked lime and the mineral potassium bisulphate – a curious mixture devised by homeopathy's founder, Samuel Hahnemann (see page 10). Homeopathic practitioners advise it for ailments of the nervous system, the mind, and the muscles, but it is also a useful first aid remedy for various types of hot or burning pains.

Typical symptoms

* Burns to the skin, especially with marked inflammation and blistering (in conjunction with appropriate first aid measures).
* Coughs, laryngitis, and hoarseness from straining or over-using the voice.
* Cystitis, particularly with involuntary passing of urine on coughing.
* Exposure to cold, dry air may worsen the symptoms.

CHAMOMILLA

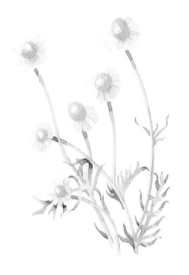

Problems helped by Chamomilla

Asthma, earache, toothache and teething, and colic. It is one of the ABC remedies for children, the others being Aconite and Belladonna.

Origin and actions

This remedy is made from the common chamomile, a member of the daisy family that grows wild over most of Europe. It strongly affects the nervous system, and should be considered only where the illness involves irritability or bad temper, especially in children.

Typical symptoms

* Irritability or bad temper.
* Excessive sensitivity to pain.
* Any childhood ailment where the child is bad-tempered or angry, especially:
* Teething pains.
* Colic where the stools smell like rotten eggs and look like slimy, chopped-up spinach.
* When pains are worse at night.
* When the temper worsens if the child is looked at, spoken to, or touched.
* When the symptoms are relieved if the child is carried or rocked.

CHINA

Problems helped by China

Fainting and collapse, also fevers.

Origin and actions

China is prepared from the dried bark of the quinaquina tree, also called Peruvian bark, cinchona, or quinine. The tree grows in the high Andes mountains of South America. This remedy affects the blood and circulation, and is usually prescribed by homeopaths on a long-term basis. It is useful for a variety of problems where the cause is extreme weakness due to loss of vital body fluids.

Typical symptoms

* Feeling faint or dizzy.
* Actual fainting or collapse, especially after dehydration (lack of water).
* Extreme weakness.
* Bleeding (haemorrhage), either from an obvious wound, or internally as from an ulcer.
* Vomiting.
* Diarrhoea.
* Fevers with profuse or drenching sweat. (A person with suspected malaria or a similar tropical disease should see a medical doctor immediately.)

Problems helped by Cocculus

Travel or motion sickness, nervous exhaustion.

Origin and actions

Prepared from the Indian cockle plant, this remedy strongly affects the central nervous system.

Typical symptoms

* Nausea, vomiting, and dizziness, as in travel sickness.
* Exhaustion and nervous stress, as when caring for a loved one, or due to lack of sleep.
* Slow reactions.

Problems helped by Coccus cacti

Coughs and whooping cough.

Origin and actions

Made from the Central American cochineal beetle, which feeds on the prickly pear cactus, this remedy affects the mucous membranes lining the throat.

Typical symptoms

* Extreme throat irritation.
* Spasms of violent coughing.
* Clear, ropey mucus that may hang from the mouth.
* Retching and vomiting.

COCCULUS and COCCUS CACTI

Problems helped by Colocynthis

Digestive upsets such as colic, diarrhoea, nausea, vomiting, and stomach pains, also period pains.

Origin and actions

Colocynthis, also known as bitter cucumber or bitter apple, is a gourd (fruit) which grows in the dry regions around the eastern Mediterranean. The remedy is prepared from the gourd's fleshy pulp. It affects the stomach and digestive tract, and also the nerves, so it is especially useful where the symptoms include irritability or even anger.

Typical symptoms

* Ailments where irritation, bad temper, or obvious anger is a predominant feature.
* Stomach or other digestive upsets, particularly where the pain is violent or cutting.
* Cramping pains in the lower abdominal or pelvic area, which may be digestive or menstrual in origin.
* Firm pressure on the affected part, or doubling up, relieves the symptoms.

COLOCYNTHIS

DIOSCOREA

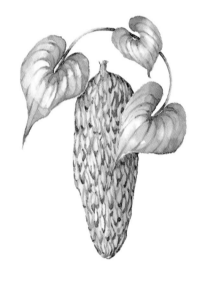

Problems helped by Dioscorea

Abdominal pains and cramps, such as colic.

Origin and actions

Dioscorea, or wild yam, is a creeping plant that grows wild in the woods and hedgerows of North America. The remedy is derived from the freshly harvested root. It acts mainly on the nerves and helps with certain types of pain in the abdominal area.

Typical symptoms

* Pains in the abdominal region, especially when these are sharp, agonizing, and "twisting" like the turn of a knife.
* Colic in babies and young children.
* Stretching the abdomen out straight, or even bending over backwards, relieves the symptoms.

DROSERA

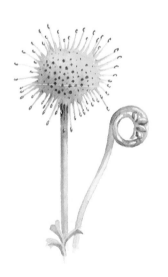

Problems helped by Drosera

Coughs and whooping cough.

Origin and actions

Drosera is the common or round-leaved sundew, a small plant that lives on heaths, marshes, and peaty bogs across the Northern Hemisphere. The glistening sticky droplets on its leaves trap insects, which the plant dissolves and absorbs. The remedy is prepared from the fresh whole plant and affects the throat, lungs, and respiratory airways. It is a major cough remedy.

Typical symptoms

* Coughs, especially when these are deep and barking.
* Coughs that are prolonged and incessant, as though they will never stop.
* Choking coughs that come in periodic fits.
* Coughs that are so severe, they may result in retching and vomiting, breathlessness, nosebleeds, and sweating.
* The symptoms are worse at night and when lying down.

Problems helped by Eupatorium

Colds and influenza.

Origin and actions

The source of Eupatorium is the aptly named herb, boneset, also called thoroughwort. The remedy is prepared from the fresh whole plant, which grows wild in damp places. It is an important treatment for colds and influenza, especially where the pain seems to have penetrated deep into the bones.

Typical symptoms

* Influenza-type symptoms, particularly where the pain seems to be deep in the bones, sometimes described as "bone-breaking".
* The muscles of the chest, back, and limbs may also feel sore and bruised.
* Nausea, with possible vomiting of bile (pale yellow, greasy fluid).
* A thirst and corresponding fever.
* A painful cough.

EUPATORIUM

Problems helped by Euphrasia

Inflammation of the eyes, and hayfever.

Origin and actions

The remedy is made from the plant euphrasia, commonly known as eyebright. It is a tall herb, with colourful flowers that open wide in the sunshine and close up on cloudy days. Euphrasia is a traditional remedy for sore and inflamed eyes, and is used by herbal as well as homeopathic practitioners.

Typical symptoms

* Eyes that feel sore and inflamed, and look red.
* The eyes water with acrid, stinging fluid.
* Hayfever symptoms, including a tickly throat, sneezing, a runny nose, and itchy, red, watering eyes – particularly where the eyes are most affected.
* Sunlight, wind, and warmth worsen the symptoms.
* The symptoms are relieved by being out in the open air.

EUPHRASIA

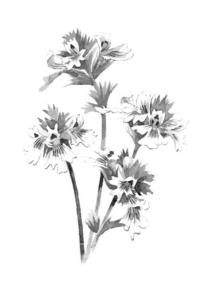

FERRUM PHOSPHORICUM
(Ferrum phos)

Problems helped by Ferrum phosphoricum

Colds and influenza, earaches, and fevers.

Origin and actions

The remedy is a chemical compound of the minerals iron and phosphorus, in the form of iron phosphate. Ferrum phosphoricum is a good all-purpose remedy for head colds, influenza, and mild fevers, especially when the symptoms come on slowly and are rather vague and ill defined.

Typical symptoms

* The symptoms develop slowly and are not clear or obvious.
* A slight temperature (about 38°C, 100°F).
* General tiredness.
* The usual symptoms of a head cold, such as a stuffed-up or runny nose, sneezing, slight feverishness, and perhaps a headache.
* Earache with violent ear pain, when the remedy indicated is Belladonna, but this has been tried and has not helped.

GELSEMIUM

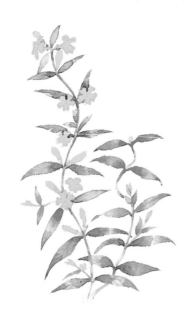

Problems helped by Gelsemium

Influenza, measles, and worry or anxiety.

Origin and actions

Gelsemium is prepared from the bark of the root of the yellow jasmine, a North American plant. The remedy acts mainly on the muscles and the nerves controlling them (the motor nerves). It is one of homeopathy's most important remedies for influenza. It can also be helpful in emotional states involving anxiety and fear of future events.

Typical symptoms

* Aching, heavy muscles with general weakness, drowsiness, fatigue, and chills.
* Shivering or trembling.
* A feeling that the mind cannot control the limbs.
* A fever with little thirst but noticeable sweating.
* A dull back-of-the-head ache.
* Drooping eyelids.
* Fear of ordeals such as exams, public speaking, or interviews.
* Anxiety after bad news.
* Sweating or urination relieve the symptoms, but emotional upsets worsen them.

Problems helped by Hamamelis

Veins that are swollen and engorged, such as haemorrhoids (piles) and varicose veins.

Origin and actions

Hamamelis is derived from witch hazel, a small tree from North America. It acts on the veins, especially in the rectal and anal area, and in the limbs. The remedy can be applied directly to the affected parts as a cream or lotion, and/or it can be taken by mouth, in the standard homeopathic pill form.

Typical symptoms

* Veins that feel bruised, painful, and sore, and that look swollen and inflamed.
* Haemorrhoids (piles), especially those which tend to bleed.
* Varicose veins that arise during pregnancy.
* Haemorrhoids (piles) that arise from pregnancy or childbirth.

HAMAMELIS

Problems helped by Hepar sulph

Coughs and croup, localized infections or septic states such as boils, abscesses, earaches, sore throats, tonsillitis, and toothache, also bronchitis.

Origin and actions

Hepar sulph is a complex mixture of the minerals calcium and sulphur, chiefly as calcium sulphide. It strongly affects the nerves, and so it is best used when the sufferer is irritable. The remedy also works well where sepsis is present.

Typical symptoms

* Irritability, and great sensitivity to external factors such as draughts, cold, noises, and being touched.
* Pains feel like sharp splinters – for example, a sore throat feels like a fishbone stuck in the throat.
* Profuse, sour-smelling sweat.
* A feeling of being chilled, which is relieved by wrapping up well, especially around the head.
* Abscesses and boils that are about to burst or discharge, and which have an offensive smell.
* A hoarse dry cough, with yellow mucus that is difficult to bring up.

HEPAR SULPH
(Hepar sulphuris calcareum)

HYPERICUM

Problems helped by Hypericum

Bruises and other injuries, especially on sensitive parts of the body.

Origin and actions

Hypericum is prepared from the herb St John's wort, using the whole fresh plant. It is mainly a remedy for injuries, with particular actions on the parts of the body rich in sensitive nerves. It can be applied directly as a cream or diluted tincture (one part of tincture in ten parts of water), or taken in the usual pill form.

Typical symptoms

* Bruising or other injury to the fingertips, toes, lips, ears, eyes, coccyx (base of the spine), and other particularly sensitive parts of the body.
* Pains may be experienced as "shooting" along the paths of the nerves.
* Apply directly to the part for minor injuries, and take by mouth as a pill for more severe injuries (along with appropriate first aid measures).

IGNATIA

Problems helped by Ignatia

Emotional upsets, shocks, and traumas.

Origin and actions

Ignatia is prepared from the bitter seeds of the St Ignatius' bean, a beautiful tree found in Eastern Asia. It is one of the most useful remedies for "emotional first aid", and it can ease many behavioural and mood problems that have an obvious emotional underlay. It may also help physical ailments that have a marked emotional or mental content.

Typical symptoms

* Sadness and depression from grief and emotional loss.
* The prolonged effects of fright, humiliation, worry, shock, and anger.
* Brooding feelings that seem to be suppressed or "locked in".
* Changeable moods, such as swinging from laughter to crying, for no obvious reason.
* Pronounced sighing.
* A feeling of a lump in the throat.
* Headaches, especially when the pain is penetrating, as if a nail is being hammered into the skull.

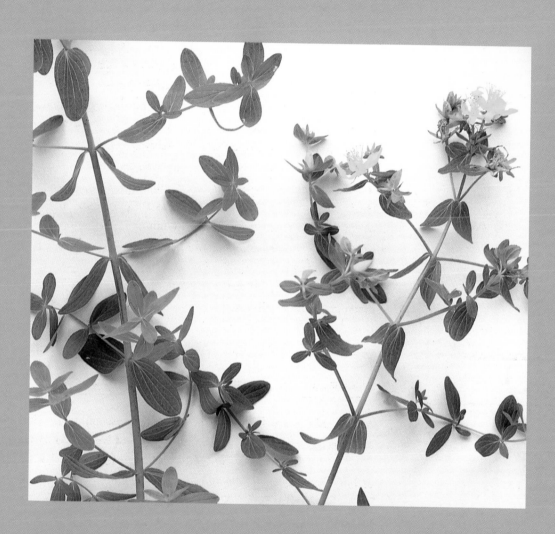

Hypericum is derived from the whole fresh plant of St John's wort (more accurately, the perforate St John's wort), a well-known herb growing across Europe and Asia. This plant is also used in herbal medicine. One explanation of its common name comes from its use during the Crusades of medieval times, to heal the wounds of the Knights of St John of Jerusalem. Another explanation is that it had witch-repelling properties and was kept in houses on the eve of the Feast of John the Baptist, during midsummer.

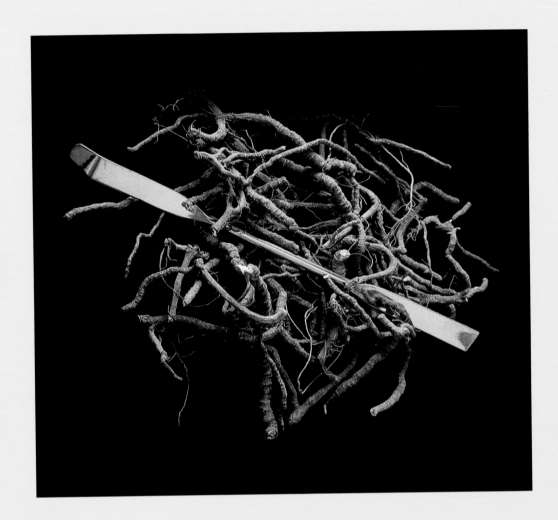

The remedy Ipecac comes from the roots and underground stems of the ipecacuanha shrub. In addition to its homeopathic uses, the roots can be ground up and prepared as a powder or syrup, which acts as an emetic to induce vomiting. This "allopathic" use in large doses is exactly the opposite of its homeopathic use in minute doses – an example of like curing like.

Problems helped by Ipecac

Nausea and vomiting, asthma, whooping cough.

Origin and actions

Ipecac is prepared from the dried root of a small South American shrub of the same name, also called ipecacuanha or the cephaelis bush. It acts mainly on the digestive tract and also on the respiratory airways. Its outstanding feature is nausea – whatever the ailment. If the illness has nausea as a predominant symptom, this remedy may help.

Typical symptoms

* Nausea (feeling sick), especially when the nausea persists even after actual vomiting, which is known as unrelieved nausea.
* Coughs, including whooping cough, which have nausea as a symptom.
* Asthma or wheeziness, when accompanied by nausea.
* Headaches, with nausea as a symptom.
* Diarrhoea, if accompanied by nausea.
* Morning sickness during pregnancy.

IPECAC (Ipecacuanha)

Problems helped by Lachesis

Sore throats, tonsillitis, women's problems such as premenstrual tension (PMT or PMS).

Origin and actions

Lachesis is prepared from the poison of the bushmaster snake. It is best prescribed by a homeopath, since it is a major constitutional and chronic, or long-term, remedy (see page 32). However it can be used at home for throat infections. Because of its emotional characteristics, it is also important for treating female problems.

Typical symptoms

* Sore throats, especially when worse on the left side, or when the soreness moves from left to right.
* Sore throats when the pain extends to the ears or neck.
* Painful swallowing, particularly when liquids are more difficult to swallow than solids.
* Symptoms that tend to be worse on waking, or when hot, or when pressure is put on the neck, chest, or waist.
* Menstrual symptoms such as cramps and irritability, which ease when the period starts.
* Hot flushes.

LACHESIS

LEDUM

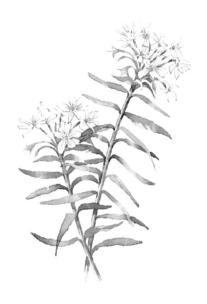

Problems helped by Ledum

Injuries, including animal bites and stings.

Origin and actions

Ledum is prepared from a small shrub called marsh tea or wild rosemary, which grows in cold bogs and marshes across Northern Europe and northern North America. It is primarily a first aid remedy, mainly used for puncture wounds, and occasionally for bloodshot eyes.

Typical symptoms

* Puncture wounds made by sharp points such as nails or wood splinters, which do not heal well and look purple and puffy.
* Insect bites and stings, which do not heal well and look purple and puffy.
* Wounds that feel cold to the touch.
* A cold compress on the wound eases the pain.
* Eye injuries when the eye becomes cold and reddened or bloodshot.

LYCOPODIUM

Problems helped by Lycopodium

Indigestion, sore throats, and many "constitutional" problems (see page 32).

Origin and actions

Lycopodium is prepared from the clubmoss plant. Homeopaths prescribe it mainly as a long-term constitutional remedy (see page 38), which acts deeply on the digestive and urinary systems. Such a deep action means that it can help a wide variety of problems, provided the symptom picture fits fairly closely.

Typical symptoms

* Heartburn.
* Flatulence and pain in the abdomen.
* Cravings for sweet things.
* Sore throats that are usually worse on the right side, or when the soreness moves from right to left.
* Low energy in the late afternoon or early evening, which can aggravate the symptoms.
* Irritability on waking.
* Gassy foods such as beans and cabbages worsen the symptoms.
* Being out in the open air relieves the symptoms.

Problems helped by Magnesia phosphorica

Colic, cramping pains such as period pains, sciatica, toothache, and earache.

Origin and actions

Magnesia phosphorica is a mineral compound of magnesium and phosphorus. It acts directly on the nerves and muscles and its chief use is for lessening or killing pain. It helps against various types of pain, but it is most effective when the symptom picture fits closely.

Typical symptoms

* Pains that are violent and paroxysmal (come in bursts or spasms).
* Pains that shoot like lightning along the nerve paths.
* Pains that are worse at night or on exposure to cold and draughts.
* Pains that are relieved by warmth (such as a hot water bottle), gentle pressure, or massage.
* In the case of cramps in the abdominal area, the pain is relieved by bending.
* When the sufferer seems to have a low pain threshold.

MERCURIUS

Problems helped by Mercurius

Infected or septic states such as boils and abscesses, sore throats and tonsillitis, earaches, toothaches, mouth ulcers, and chickenpox and mumps.

Origin and actions

Mercurius is prepared from liquid metal mercury (quicksilver) or its complex salt ammonium nitrate of mercury. It strongly affects the body's glands and their secretions. It comes into its own when sepsis has set in, and an infected area has turned septic or "gone bad".

Typical symptoms

* Swollen glands.
* Increased saliva, which is often even more plentiful at night.
* Profuse sweating.
* A tongue which is flabby and yellowish, and which may show the imprint of the teeth.
* Increased thirst.
* The breath, secretions, and discharges have offensive odours.
* Any discharges may be blood-streaked.
* A metallic taste in the mouth.
* Emotional exhaustion, with irritability and restlessness.

NATRUM MURIATICUM (Nat mur)

Problems helped by Natrum muriaticum

Grief and similar emotional problems, including resentment.

Origin and actions

This remedy is basically sodium chloride, or common salt. It is a major constitutional remedy (see pages 32 and 40) and works deeply on the emotions. Natrum muriaticum can aid many chronic or long-term problems, if the symptoms and personality features fit. On a physical level, it affects the body's water balance.

Typical symptoms

* Feelings of grief, resentment, or humiliation, which tend to become suppressed, held back, or "bottled up".
* Continuous crying – or, conversely, almost no tears when crying would be expected.
* Enjoyment of being alone.
* Dislike of being consoled.
* A very sensitive nature, tending to over-react.
* Cravings for salt and salty foods.
* Headaches from the sun.
* Cold sores (oral herpes) especially around the mouth.

NATRUM SULPHURICUM (Nat sulph)

Problems helped by Natrum sulphuricum

Asthma that is made worse by damp conditions.

Origin and actions

Natrum sulphuricum is made from sodium sulphate, a mineral compound of sodium and sulphur, also known as Glauber's salts. It has effects on the liver and the head, as well as the respiratory system. It tends to be most useful for people who are badly affected by the damp, or whose symptoms worsen in damp conditions.

Typical symptoms

* Acute asthmatic breathing, that is, sudden attacks of wheeziness, breathlessness, and even panting.
* Asthma-type attacks that are brought on by the damp or wet weather.
* Asthma that is often worse in the early morning.
* Asthma or wheeziness that follows a cold or great exertion.
* Ailments that may date back to a previous head injury.

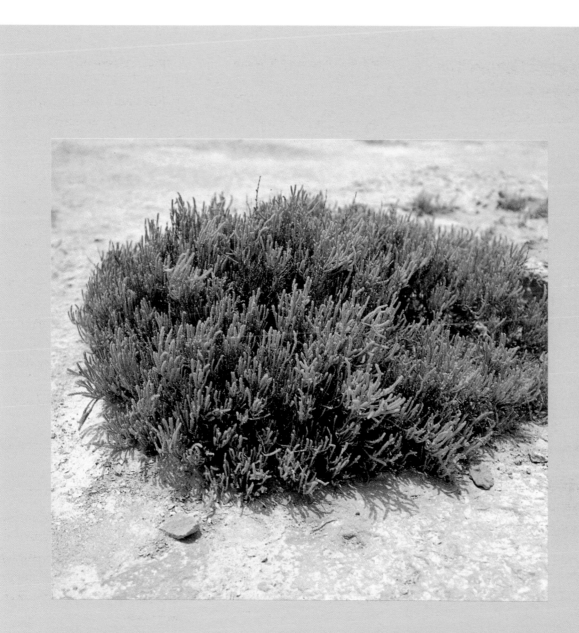

Life began in the salty water of the sea. Common sea salt – sodium chloride – is essential to life, regulating the fluids and the flow of vital minerals throughout the body. Plants of the coastal saltmarsh, such as glasswort, take up the salt and are rich sources of sodium and chlorides.

NUX VOMICA

Problems helped by Nux vomica

Indigestion, nausea, vomiting, hangover headaches, colds, and influenza.

Origin and actions

Nux vomica is derived from the seeds of the strychnine-containing poison nut tree, which grows in Eastern Asia. It is a major remedy for first aid situations, especially those affecting the digestive system. It is also a very important constitutional and chronic, or long term, remedy (see page 32).

Typical symptoms

* Nausea or vomiting.
* Digestive problems from too much rich food and alcohol.
* Hangover headaches caused by too much alcohol.
* The urge to pass a stool (bowel motion), with no or unsatisfactory results.
* Alternating diarrhoea and constipation.
* When food lies like a heavy load or weight in the stomach.
* Watery, sour heartburn.
* A very sensitive, irritable, and impatient temperament.
* A tendency to insomnia.

PHOSPHORUS

Problems helped by Phosphorus

Nausea, vomiting, diarrhoea, nosebleeds, and other minor bleeding, and "constitutional" problems (see page 32).

Origin and actions

The mineral phosphorus is an essential constituent of the body, particularly the bones. As an important constitutional remedy, it can help many problems where the personality and symptoms agree. It has special effects on the digestive tract and respiratory airways.

Typical symptoms

* This remedy is best chosen by matching the symptoms and personality picture as described on page 42.
* In particular, phosphorus may suit people who are normally lively, open, and friendly, but who are also occasionally nervous and anxious, perhaps needing reassurance from others.

Problems helped by Phytolacca

Sore throats and tonsillitis, also mastitis and other nipple or breast problems.

Origin and actions

Phytolacca is prepared from the small shrub of the same name, also known as poke root, that grows across the Northern Hemisphere. The parts used are the fresh leaves or ripe berries. The remedy affects mainly the body's glands and glandular tissues, including the tonsils and breasts (mammary glands).

Typical symptoms

* Sore throats where the back of the mouth and throat look very dark and "angry".
* Sore throats where the pain feels like a hot ball and is worse on swallowing.
* A sore throat that feels better after cold drinks, but worse in warm conditions.
* Pain in both ears, which is made worse by swallowing.
* Cracked or sore nipples.
* Swollen, tender breasts that feel hard and "stony", and which may occur when breastfeeding.

PHYTOLACCA

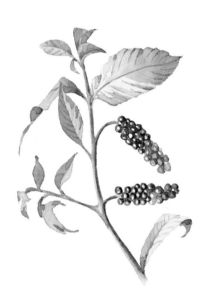

PODOPHYLLUM

Problems helped by Podophyllum

Diarrhoea and other gastro-intestinal upsets.

Origin and actions

Podophyllum is derived from a North American herb known as the May apple or mandrake. It can be made from the whole fresh plant, or from the ripe fruit, or from the root after the fruit has fallen. The remedy chiefly affects the duodenum and the rest of the small intestine, and the large intestine, especially its last part, the rectum.

Typical symptoms

* Diarrhoea which is explosive and mixed with gas.
* Diarrhoea which is extraordinarily profuse and watery.
* Diarrhoea that gushes out painlessly.
* Suitable for the bilious or liverish constitution, especially when the liver area (in the upper abdomen) is sore and painful.

PULSATILLA

Problems helped by Pulsatilla

Asthma, chickenpox, mumps, earache, eye problems, teething, and other childhood problems, and also menstrual problems.

Origin and actions

Pulsatilla, made from the pasque flower, is an essential part of a basic homeopathy kit, especially the first aid kit. It is a major constitutional remedy (see pages 32 and 42). If the emotional symptoms fit, it can be very helpful, even if the physical problem does not correspond.

Typical symptoms

* Emotions and moods that are always changing.
* Physical symptoms that constantly change.
* A tendency to be weepy and sensitive, and to cling or hold on.
* A sympathetic and gentle nature.
* Little or no thirst with most ailments.
* Yellow-green discharges.
* The symptoms are relieved by cool, fresh air and the company of others.
* Rich, fatty foods aggravate the symptoms.

RHUS TOX

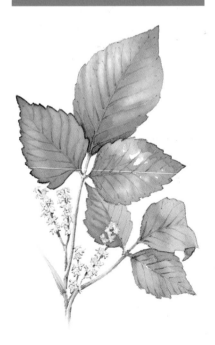

Problems helped by Rhus tox

Chickenpox, mumps, shingles, sprains and strains and joint pains.

Origin and actions

Rhus tox is prepared from the North American rambling plant, poison ivy. It is an important first aid remedy for sprains, strains, swollen joints, and similar injuries. It can also help many other problems, provided the symptom picture fits fairly closely.

Typical symptoms

* Extreme restlessness.
* Stiffness in the joints, that eases after gentle movement.
* Swollen glands.
* A rash which is extremely itchy and red.
* A thirst for large quantities of water or milk.
* The symptoms are relieved by warmth and massage.
* The symptoms are worsened by cold, dampness, and over-exertion.

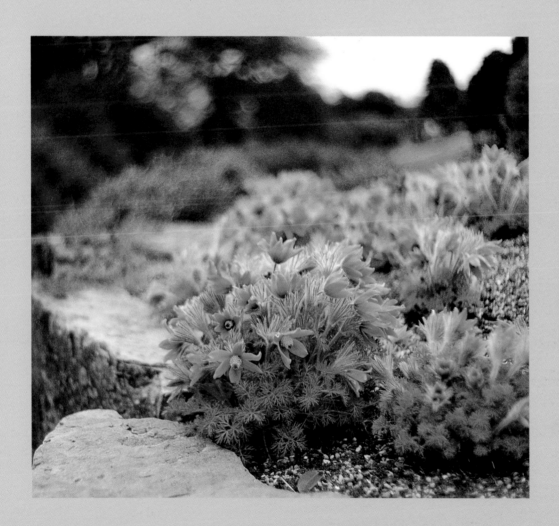

The remedy Pulsatilla comes from the pasque flower, also known as the wind flower. This is a plant of the anemone family, with purple, bell-like flowers. Pulsatilla is sometimes called the weather-cock remedy, since people who benefit from it have ever-changing feelings and moods.

RUMEX

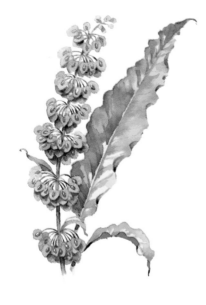

Problems helped by Rumex

Coughs, especially ticklish, persistent coughing.

Origin and actions

Rumex is prepared from the fresh roots of the plant called yellow or curled dock. This is a wayside weed growing in North America and Europe. The remedy has marked effects on the nerves, and also on the mucous membranes which line the lower throat and larynx.

Typical symptoms

* A dry, teasing cough, that comes from constant irritation, and which is often worse at night.
* A cough that is triggered or aggravated by inhaling cold air, which gives the feeling of a feather tickling the throat.
* Warmth and covering the mouth relieve the symptoms.

RUTA

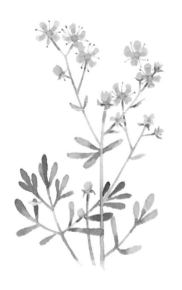

Problems helped by Ruta

Bruises, eye strains, and sprains and strains affecting the muscles and joints.

Origin and actions

Ruta is prepared from the herb rue, which has been treasured through the ages for its medicinal properties. The remedy has effects on the joints, tendons, cartilages, and the periosteum (the membrane that covers the bones). It is also valued for its first aid qualities and its action on tired eyes.

Typical symptoms

* Painful bruises affecting the bones.
* Strains to the tendons or joints, especially in the ankles and wrists.
* Aching with restlessness.
* Cold and damp conditions make the symptoms worse.
* Sensations of being over-strained and stiff.
* Lower back pain that feels better when lying down.
* Eye strains, particularly when accompanied by dim vision.

SABADILLA

Problems helped by Sabadilla

Hayfever and other irritations of the nose, where sneezing is the worst complaint.

Origin and actions

Sabadilla is prepared from the seeds of the cebadilla or asagraea plant, from Mexico. These seeds were once used for destroying body parasites such as lice and worms. The homeopathic remedy is of course much gentler. It affects particularly the mucous membranes lining the nasal cavities.

Typical symptoms

* Violent sneezing, usually in spasms.
* An itching nose.
* The nose feels stuffy and dry, yet it still has a runny discharge.
* Sensitivity to pollen, dust, and other small inhaled particles, and even the scent of flowers.
* Watering eyes.
* The symptoms may improve in the open air and when it is warm, and worsen in the cold.

SARSAPARILLA

Problems helped by Sarsaparilla

Chiefly cystitis.

Origin and actions

Sarsaparilla is derived from the roots of a North American plant of the same name, sometimes called smilax or wild liquorice. The remedy acts primarily on the parts of the urinary and genital (sexual) systems. Its most important use is against cystitis, which is inflammation of the bladder lining, usually associated with bacterial infection.

Typical symptoms

* Symptoms of cystitis, mainly a burning pain on urination, and a frequent urge to urinate, but little urine is passed.
* Urination is slow, and the pain is particularly bad at the end.
* The pain can be so bad that you may actually scream with agony.

SEPIA

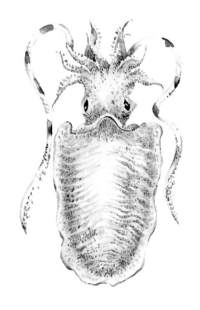

Problems helped by Sepia

Chiefly female ailments, including menstrual and PMT problems.

Origin and actions

Sepia is a remedy derived from the ink of a sea-dwelling mollusc, the cuttlefish. It is not exclusively a woman's remedy. But it does have a powerful effect on the female reproductive system, and it can be helpful in all stages of a woman's life – from puberty through to the menopause, and including pregnancy and menstrual problems.

Typical symptoms

* Emotional indifference to life, even to loved ones.
* Irritable, easily offended, and stuck in depression.
* Nausea and sensitivity to smells such as food being cooked.
* Morning sickness.
* Feelings of lower abdominal or pelvic prolapse, as if the internal organs might drop down.
* Irregular periods.
* Hot flushes.
* Strenuous exercise relieves the symptoms.

SILICA

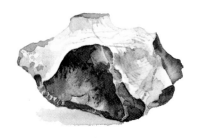

Problems helped by Silica

Abscesses, wounds that are slow to heal, toothache and earache, and similar localized infections.

Origin and actions

Silica is a mineral prepared from sand or flint rock. Homeopaths tend to use it more for long-term prescriptions than for everyday ailments. However it can be very useful for treating pus-filled or suppurating wounds, since it encourages the body to expel diseased tissues, or to break down and reabsorb them.

Typical symptoms

* Small-scale infections that seem to be turning septic or putrid, rather than healing.
* Abscesses that linger without coming to a head, as in some types of toothaches.
* Foreign bodies such as splinters, pieces of grit, or fragments of glass, that the body needs to expel.
* This remedy is especially suitable for symptoms that are slow to heal, or for people who feel the cold, or who lack stamina or vitality.

SPONGIA

Problems helped by Spongia

Coughs and croup, and various throat and larynx (voice-box) ailments, such as sore throats and laryngitis.

Origin and actions

The lightly roasted and powdered skeleton of the common sponge, a simple sea animal, produces the remedy Spongia. It has strong effects on the airways and respiratory system, and so is excellent for coughs, sore throats, and similar problems of the respiratory tract.

Typical symptoms

* A dry and hollow cough that sounds barking or hacking, and that comes in spasms or fits.
* A cough that rasps heavily, so that it sounds like a saw being pushed and pulled through a wooden board.
* Tickling, dryness, and feelings of constriction in the throat.
* Any cough is usually worse before midnight, and improved after eating or drinking, especially warm drinks.
* Exercise or great activity worsens the symptoms.

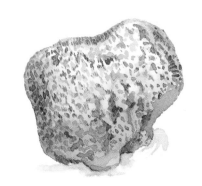

STAPHYSAGRIA

Problems helped by Staphysagria

Styes and eye infections, the after-effects of surgery, and emotional stresses and upsets.

Origin and actions

Staphysagria is prepared from the larkspur flower, a member of the delphinium family. It suits sensitive people who suppress their feelings and suffer in silence, or who boil over with indignation. This can be a remedy for cuts and wounds, especially when linked to feelings of indignation or humiliation.

Typical symptoms

* Styes or eye inflammation that may result from overwork, stress, or fatigue.
* Cuts and wounds from surgery, such as episiotomy or dental treatment, especially when these are slow to heal.
* Emotional stress and other complaints that follow suppressed feelings of anger, grief, or humiliation.
* Especially suitable if there are feelings of being used or manipulated.

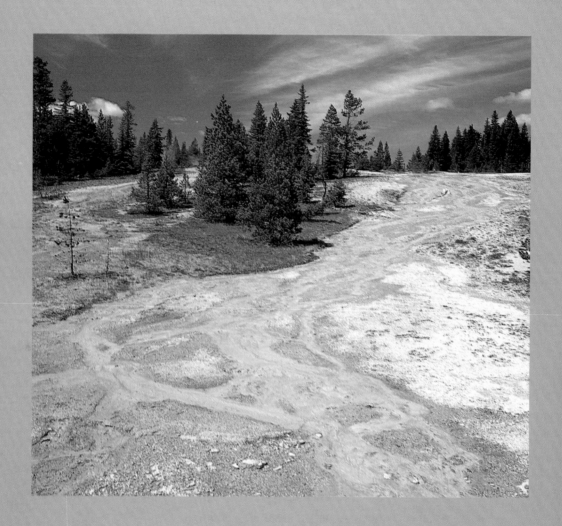

Sulphur is present in many natural places, from the choking fumes of a volcano, to the stinking odours of bubbling marsh gas, to the invigorating aromas of spa mineral waters. This yellowish elemental substance has been used for healing purposes for more than 5,000 years.

SULPHUR

Problems helped by Sulphur

Sulphur is a major constitutional and children's remedy (see pages 32 and 46). It can help a large number of problems if the person is of the Sulphur type.

Origin and actions

Sulphur is a natural element that in its raw state looks like yellowish chalk. It is a very deep-acting remedy on any part of the body. It helps to remove poisons and toxins and bring them to the surface, hence its association with skin problems.

Typical symptoms

The personality or constitutional type is likely to be as important as the symptoms and ailment. The main personality features are as follows (see also page 42):
* People who live mainly in their minds and heads, without noticing their surroundings.
* People who have a low point around 11am, when a snack may be necessary to boost the body's energy levels.
* People who are "warm-blooded" and who do not seem to feel the cold.
* People who have a sweet tooth.

SYMPHYTUM

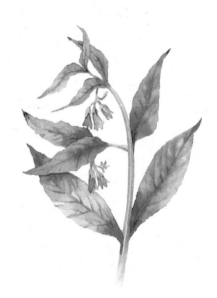

Problems helped by Symphytum

Fractures (broken bones) and eye injuries.

Origin and actions

Symphytum is derived from the herb common comfrey, also known as knitbone, which grows wild in Europe. The remedy is made from the whole fresh plant. Its main use is to help heal broken bones, but it also has healing effects on the eye.

Typical symptoms

* Bone breaks or fractures. Once a fracture has been reduced or "set" with the bones back in their normal position, Symphytum speeds up the knitting or fusing together of the bones. It must be used after the fracture is reduced, or the bones may heal out of alignment.
* Injuries to the eye ball, such as being hit by a hard object, like a tennis ball.

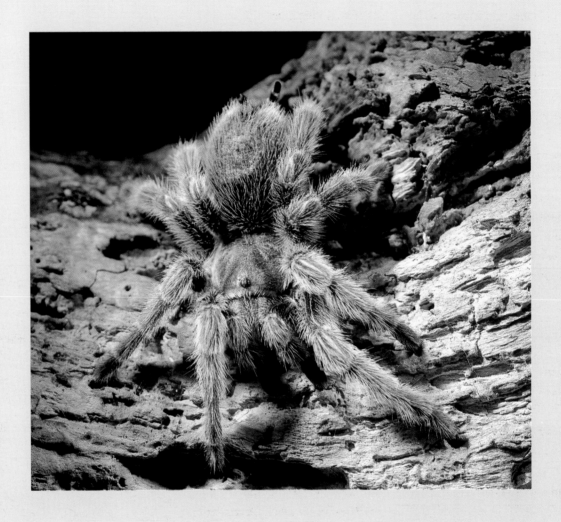

The fearsome-looking tarantula spider has a bite that is not particularly painful at first, but soon becomes extremely stinging and painful. The remedy Tarentula cubensis is prepared from one type of tarantula, from Cuba.

TABACUM

Problems helped by Tabacum

Travel or motion sickness, in boats, planes, trains, cars, and even on fairground rides.

Origin and actions

Tabacum is a remedy derived from the tobacco plant. In homeopathic doses, it can cure certain symptoms produced by smoking tobacco. These symptoms are produced by the chemical nicotine in tobacco smoke, and they are similar to those experienced in travel or motion sickness.

Typical symptoms

* A deathly pale face and overwhelming nausea.
* The nausea may be followed by actual vomiting.
* Profuse sweating.
* A sinking feeling in the stomach.
* A headache that is accompanied by severe nausea.
* Fresh, cool air relieves the symptoms.

TARENTULA CUBENSIS

Problems helped by Tarentula cubensis

Serious boils, abscesses, and ulcers, and similar eruptions.

Origin and actions

The venomous Cuban tarantula spider provides the remedy Tarentula cubensis. The symptoms helped by the remedy resemble those produced by the spider's bite.

Typical symptoms

* In the first stages, there seems to be little wrong, but the symptoms rapidly worsen. (Similarly, the spider's bite is initially not very painful.)
* Boils and similar infected or septic conditions, particularly when these incubate and develop slowly, and then come to a head and mature rapidly and alarmingly.
* The affected part is hard and purple, with a terrible burning pain.
* The area around the boil swells and reddens.

URTICA

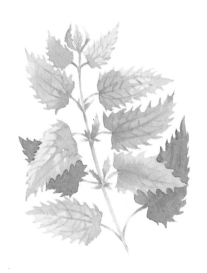

Problems helped by Urtica

Burns, insect bites and stings, hives, and prickly heat.

Origin and actions

The herb urtica is better known as the small stinging nettle. The fresh plant in flower yields a useful remedy. In particular, it can help many skin problems which resemble the well-known rash caused by the nettle. It can also increase the supply of milk in breastfeeding mothers.

Typical symptoms

* Minor burns, bites, stings, and skin rashes.
* Symptoms that arise from allergic reactions, such as eating shellfish.
* Urticaria or similar complaints with stinging or burning pains in the skin.
* Breastfeeding problems where the supply of milk is lacking.

VERATRUM ALBUM

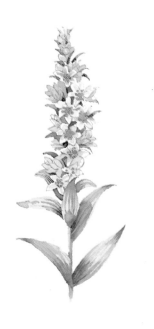

Problems helped by Veratrum album

Chiefly diarrhoea and vomiting, and other digestive disturbances.

Origin and actions

Veratrum album is prepared from the rootstock of the herb white hellebore. Homeopaths use it widely for treating chronic or long-term ailments, but it is also a well known remedy for "violent eruptions" at both ends of the digestive tract. It is therefore a major remedy for illnesses such as cholera and dysentery.

Typical symptoms

* Violent and continual vomiting and/or diarrhoea (in conjunction with first aid and medical treatment).
* Extreme chilliness and weakness.
* A thirst for ice-cold water, which sometimes seems to be unquenchable, yet the water may be vomited straight back.
* Profuse, cold sweats, especially on the forehead.
* A desire for sour or sharp fruits, lemons, salt, and ice.
* The symptoms worsen in cold conditions.

VERBASCUM

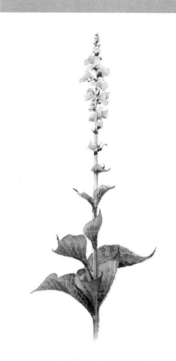

Problems helped by Verbascum

Earaches of all kinds, both in children and adults.

Origin and actions

Verbascum is normally used as an oil, which has been prepared from the plant variously known as common mullein, great mullein, or Aaron's rod. This grows in many places across North America and Europe. A few drops of the warmed oil placed in the ear have a very soothing effect.

Typical symptoms

* Any earaches.
* If Verbascum oil is not to hand, a few drops of olive oil in the ear may be soothing.

RESCUE REMEDY

Problems helped by Rescue remedy

Crises and shocks of various kinds.

Origin and actions

The Rescue remedy is not a true homeopathic remedy. It comes from the system of healing and medicine called the Bach Flower remedies. The Rescue remedy is a combination of five of these flower remedies. It is included here because it can be used in conjunction with any other homeopathic remedy.

Typical symptoms

* Any extreme crisis or shock, either mental or physical, in conjunction with homeopathic remedies and other treatments, as appropriate.

The Home Homeopathy Kit

Of the 60 or so homeopathic remedies described in this book, some are virtually essential for your home remedy kit. Others have more specialized or restricted applications, and they may be used once in a lifetime, or perhaps not at all.

About 20 remedies and five creams or tinctures should suffice for a basic kit. Those on the right are likely to be the most useful.

For advice on handling and storing remedies, see below and page 51.

The basic kit

Pills (6C or 30C)

Aconite	Hypericum
Apis	Ignatia
Arnica	Ledum
Arsenicum	Lycopodium
Belladonna	Mercurius
Bryonia	Nux vomica
Chamomilla	Phosphorus
Ferrum phosphoricum	Pulsatilla
(Ferrum phos)	Rhus tox
Gelsemium	Ruta
Hepar sulph	

Creams and tinctures

Arnica cream, for bruises
Calendula (or Hypercal) cream, for cuts and sores
Euphrasia tincture, which must be diluted for eyes

Rescue cream (from the Bach Flower remedies system)
Urtica (or Burn combination) cream, for burns, scalds, bites, and stings

Other essentials

In addition to the basic homeopathy kit above, the well-stocked first aid cupboard should contain Rescue remedy (see page 137). Ensure all remedy bottles have their lids securely tightened.

Other useful items include bandages, sticking plasters, tweezers (forceps) and round-ended scissors.

All of these the items should be kept in a secure box with a lid. Place the box in a cool, dry place, well away from strong smells such as camphor, eucalyptus, or perfumes. It is also best to avoid vibrations and radiation from TV sets, computers, and similar equipment. Remedies should last indefinitely under these conditions. Keep the kit well out of reach of children, even though homeopathic remedies are very safe.

Extra remedies

Add to the basic kit according to the needs of your household. For example, if you have a colicky child, you may want to add Colocynthis or Magnesia phosphorica. Eupatorium can be good for bone-aching influenza. If haemorrhoids are a regular problem, then include Hamamelis cream and/or Aesculus cream. Consider Drosera, Spongia, and Rumex if someone is always getting coughs.

Constitutional remedies

You may be able to identify the constitutional type of your child yourself, using the descriptions given in this book, and noting the effects that the remedies have on the child in times of illness. Then keep a stock of this particular remedy.

You could consult a homeopath for an interview and advice about possible constitutional prescribing for yourself and other adults, and of course for children.

Pill potencies

For home prescribing, use pills of 6th (6C) or 30th (30C) potency. With 6C you will probably have to repeat the doses more often.

See pages 14 and 16-17 for further information.

Where to obtain remedies

Health stores, health food shops, and some pharmacies and chemists may stock the most common 6C remedies. However, these may be in cartons, which can be bulky to store.

It is probably most convenient, especially if you want to buy a number of remedies, to contact one of the major homeopathic pharmacies listed on the following page. Most of them can supply the remedies in a useful container, by mail order. They will also accept credit card payments or payment on delivery, and they usually have a have a 24-hour answering service.

Alternatively, you could consult your telephone directory for a suitable local store or shop, or contact a practitioner (see below).

Remedies are inexpensive.

Finding a practitioner – The Society of Homeopaths

As with any therapist, word of mouth recommendation is often best. If you cannot find a homeopathic practitioner in your area, contact:
The Society of Homeopaths
2 Artizan Road
Northampton NN1 4HV
Telephone 0604 21400
This is the main organization for training and registering qualified

homeopaths. They can offer help and advice, and put you in contact with local practitioners.

The British Homeopathic Association

Some orthodox medical doctors have completed a postgraduate course in homeopathy, in addition to their medical training. A few may offer homeopathy under the National Health Service. For more information, contact:
The British Homeopathic Association
27A Devonshire Street
London W1N 1RJ
Telephone 071 935 2163

Resources

Pharmacies

Helios Homeopathic Pharmacy
97 Camden Road
Tonbridge Wells
Kent TN1 2QR
Telephone 0892 537254/536393

Nelson's Pharmacy
73 Duke Street
London W1M 6BY
Telephone 071 629 3118

Ainsworths Pharmacy
38 New Cavendish Street
London W1M 7LH
Telephone 071 935 5330

Training courses

Some local education authorities run classes in homeopathy. These can be an excellent practical introduction to the subject. If you are interested in professional training, contact one of the dozen or so colleges in the UK. They offer a four-year part-time course, and in some cases a three-year full-time one. For information:

The Society of Homeopaths
2 Artizan Road
Northampton NN1 4HV
Telephone 0604 21400

Books, bookshops, and magazines

Many books on homeopathy are available, although most are for the professional and hard to find. Some of the general titles are:

Homeopathy: Medicine of the New Man
George Vithoulkis
(Thorsons, 1985)

Magic of the Minimum Dose
Dorothy Shepherd
(CW Daniel, 1964)

More Magic of the Minimum Dose
Dorothy Shepherd
(CW Daniel, 1974)

A Physicians Posy
Dorothy Shepherd
(CW Daniel, 1969)

If you want to know more about the remedies you need a good Materia Medica. Two excellent versions, written for the professional but in an accessible style, are:

Homeopathic Drug Pictures
Margaret Tyler
(CW Daniel, 1970)

Studies of Homeopathic Remedies
Douglas Gibson
(Beaconsfield, 1987)

A good book on nutrition can be invaluable. A very useful one is:

Nutritional Medicine
Alan Stewart and Stephen Davies
(Pan, 1987)

If you have trouble locating these books, try:

Watkins Bookshop
19 Cecil Court
Charing Cross Road
London WC2N 4EZ
Telephone 071 836 2182

Minerva Books Mail Order Service
6 Bothwell Street
London W6 8DY
Telephone 071 385 1361

There is also a fascinating monthly magazine containing valuable information on how medical doctors practise, with details of the drugs used and their side-effects, plus ideas about alternative and less invasive methods of treatment:

What Doctors Don't Tell You
4 Wallace Road
London N1 2BG
Telephone 071 354 4592

Acknowledgements

Photographic credits
Gaia Books 9, 19, 23, 29, 33, 54, 69, 85, 97, 117
Tony Morrison 13
Ellen Moorcraft 37, 39, 41, 43, 45, 47
Steve Gregory/Bruce Coleman 49
Clem Haagner/Ardea London Ltd 60
Geoff Dore/Bruce Coleman 65
D.Yendall/Natural Science Photos 79
Michael Fogden/Oxford Scientific Films 82
Richard Revels/Natural Science Photos 105
Deni Bown/Oxford Scientific Films 108
Edward Parker 118
Michael Jones/ A-Z Botanical Collection Ltd 123
Heather Angel 127
Stan Osolinski/Oxford Scientific Films 132
John Mason/Ardea 134

Gaia would like to extend particular thanks to the following people:
Winnie Appleby, Sam and Matty Barnet, Lizzie Mason, Sadie Wickwar, and Robert Whitworth for their work as models.
Dr. Brian Kaplan for checking the text.
Katherine Pate and Jane Parker for proofreading the text.
Mary Warren for preparing the Index.

INDEX

Bold type indicates main entry
Italic type indicates illustration

A
Aaron's rod 137
abdominal pains 112
abscesses 94, 115, 121, 130
accidents 53, **85-95**,
acne 74
Aconite 55, 58, 73, 75, 77, **100**
    for coughs 56, 72
    for fear 83, 89, 90, 92
    in fevers 57, 76
acute illnesses 15, 51
Acquired Immune Deficiency Syndrome
(AIDS) 27
Aesculus 29, 63, **100**
allergies 25-8, 53, 74, 75, **79-81**, 101
    see also asthma; food; hayfever
Allium cepa 55, 81, 101
anaemia 63, **68**
anger 84, 111
animals 27
    see also bites and stings
antibiotics 20, 22
antidotes 51, 59
Antimonium tartaricum (Ant tart) 71, **101**
antiseptics 86
anus 100
anxiety **83**, 102, 103, 114
Apis 57, 58, 76, 77, 86, **102**
Argentum nitricum (Arg nit) 61, 83, **102**
Arnica 86, 90, 91, 92, **103**
    as cream 16, 87, 88, 93
arsenic 103
Arsenicum album (Ars alb) 83, 86, **103**
    colds 55, 57, 81
    diarrhoea 61, 63
    respiratory 70, 80
arteriosclerosis 20
asagraea plant 129
aspirin 22
asthma 28, 40, 70, **80**, 103, 119, 126

B
Bach flower remedies 51, 90, 137
bacterial infections 78
bad breath 57, 77, 94
bee's sting venom 102
behavioural problems 116
Belladonna 8, 10, 58, 68, 71, 77, **104**, *105*, 114
    fevers 55, 57, 73, 76
    infections 86, 89, 94
    bites and stings 86, 102, 107, 120, 136
bitter apple or cucumber 111
bladder problems 66, 107
bleeding 88, 92, 93, 94, 110, 115
    see also nosebleeds
blistering 87, 109
bloating 102

blood circulation 110
bloody discharges 63
body fluids 110
body temperature 56, 58
boils **86**, 104, 115, 121, 135
    on eyes **89**
boneset 54, 113
"bottling up" 84, 89, 122
bowels 100
breastfeeding problems 26, 65, **68**, 125, 136
breast problems 68, 125
breathing problems 56, 101
breathlessness 70, 112
British Homeopathy Association, The 139
bronchitis 104, 115
bruises 86, **87**, 91, 103, 107, 116, 128
Bryonia 63, 68, 74, 76, 77, 78, **104**
    colds 55, 56, 57
    injuries 91, 93
burns 87, 107, 136
bushmaster snake 119

C
Calcarea carbonica (Calc carb) 32, *33*, 37, 68, **106**
    constitutional type 35-7
Calcarea phosphorica (Calc phos) 91, **106**
calcium phosphate 106
calcium sulphide 115
Calendula 18, *19*, **107**
    cream 16, 71, 74, 103
    cream or tincture 86, 87, 88, 93
calming 93
camphor 51, 59
Cantharis 66, 86, 87, **107**
Carbo vegetablis (Carbo veg) 90, *108*, **109**
cartilages 128
Causticum 66, 87, **109**
cebadilla plant 129
central nervous system 111
cephaelis bush 119
chamomile 110
Chamomilla 69, 70, 73, 75,77, 80, 94, **110**
charcoal 109
chickenpox 27, 71, 101, 104, 121, 126
children
    ailments 27, 48, 53, 56, **69-78**, 106
    behaviour and emotions 75, 110
    constitutional types **32-47**
    emergencies 70, 72
    fears and worries 36, 38, 40, 42, 44, 46
    prescribing for 32-47, 106, 133
chills 114
China (China officinalis) 90, 92, **110**
cholera 136
chronic illnesses 15
cinchona 110
cirrhosis 20
clamminess 101
"clean tongue" 50, 51
clubmoss 120

Cocculus 83, 95, **111**
Coccus cacti 78, **111**
cochineal beetle 111
colds 53, 100, 103, 104, 106, 114, 124
cold sores 40, 122
colic 62, 72, 110, 111, 112, 121
collapse **90**, 109, 110
Colocynthis 60, 61, 63, 67, 72, **111**
comfrey 8, 133
common ailments
    index 53
    treatments **48-95**
common mullein 52, 137
common sponge 131
compresses 86, 88, 89, 91, 102, 120
conjunctivitis 89
constipation 106
constitutions 16-17
    remedies 34, 133
    types **32-47**
coughs 36, **56**, 100, 104, 106, 109, 111, 112, 115, 119, 128, 131
    see also croup; whooping cough
crises 137
croup 56, **72**, 100, 115, 131
cuts **88**, 107, 131
cuttlefish 130
cystitis 65, **66**, 107, 109, 129

D
deadly nightshade 8-10, 104
dehydration 61, 63, 87
dental treatment 93, 94
depression 84, 116
diabetes 51
diarrhoea **61**, 83, 102, 110, 111, 119, 124, 125, 136
diet 23, 24-5, 28, 30, 63, 68
digestive problems 11, 46, 53, 60, **61-4**, 103, 111, 124
digestive tract 119, 124
dilated pupils 58, 76
dilutions 12-14, 51, 96
Dioscorea 72, **112**
discharges 86, 89, 94, 126
    bloody 63, 121
    nasal 59, 73, 81, 103
diseases 25-6, 49
    see also specific ailments
dizziness 109
dosages 35, 50, 51
Drosera 56, 78, 79, **112**
drowsiness 101, 102, 114
drugs 20, 22-4, 28, 51
dysentery 136

E
earache 52, 63, 100, 104, 114, 115, 121, 126, 130, 137
    in children **73**
eczema **74**
electromagnetic radiations 20, 51

emergencies 51, 53, 80, **85-95**
emotional upsets 53, 102, 114, 116, 122, 130, 131
    in children **75**, **82-3**
epilepsy 51
essential nutrients 24, 25, 28-30
eucalyptus 51, 59
Eupatorium *54* 55, 63, **113**
Euphrasia 74, 81, 88, 89, **113**
exercise 30
exhaustion 111, 121
extroverts 46
eyebright 113
eyelids, soreness 89
eye problems 100, 102, 113, 126, 129, 131
    inflammation **89**, 113
    injuries **88**, 120, 133
eyestrain **88**, 128

F
fainting **90**, 109, 110
fatigue 114
Ferrum phosphoricum (Ferrum phos) 55, 56, 68, 73, **114**
fevers 15
    in children 36, 53, 55, 56, **57**
    remedies 100, 102, 104, 106, 110, 114
first aid 17, 85, 90, 91, 116
    remedies 107, 109, 124
flatulence 38, 62, 109, 120
food 25, 28, 61, 62, 63, 75
    see also diet
food poisoning 103
foreign bodies 73, 89, 130
fractures **91**, 106, 133
fright 61, 75, 90, 102, 116

G
Gandhi, Mahatma 48
gargling 58
Gelsemium 55, 57, 59, 74, 75, 76, 83, **114**
genitals 129
german measles (rubella) **74**
gingivitis 94
glands, swollen 57, 59, **77**, 106, 121, 125
glasswort *123*
Glauber's salts 122
grief 83, **84**, 116, 122
growing pains 106
guide to remedies **96-139**
gums, inflammation 94

H
Haemorrhage *see* bleeding
haemorrhoids 29, 100, 115
Hahnemann, Samuel 10-14, 18, 96
Hamamelis 63, 115
hangovers 62, 124
hayfever 40, **81**, 103, 113
headaches 104, 114, 116, 122
    in children 56, 57, 63, 106
    with nausea 119, 124, 135

healing energy 31
heartburn 62, 120, 124
Hepar sulph 56, 58, 72, 73, 94, **115**
herbs 51
hiccups 62
Hippocrates 10
hives 136
hoarseness 109
home prescribing 16-17, 20, 34, 139
    kit **138-9**
homeopathy
    history 10-15
    principles 8-10, 17, 50-1
horse chestnut 29, 101
hot flushes 66, 119, 130
Human Immunodeficiency Virus (HIV) 27, 30
Hypercal 86, 87, 88
Hypericum 87, 88, 93, *117*, **116**
hysteria 83, 84

I
Ignatia 75, 83, 84, 90, 92, **116**
imbalance suppression 74
immune system 20, 22, 26-31, 32, 80
impatience 124
indecision 44
Index of Common Ailments 53
Index of Remedies 99
Indian cockle plant 111
indifference 67
indigestion 62, 120, 124
indignation 131
individuality 72, 78
infants 72, 78
infections 53, 77, 78, 101, 107, 115
infectious diseases 25-7, 71, 74, **76**
inflammation 59, 73, **89**, 94, 113
    remedies 101, 102, 104, 107, 109
influenza 54, **55**, 100, 103, 104, 114, 124
injuries 15, 53, **85-95**, 116, 120
    eyes **88**, 133
insect bites **86**, 107, 136
insomnia 102, 124
insulin 22
interaction of treatments 51
intestines 62
Ipecac (Ipecacuanha) 63, 70, 78, 80, *118*, 119
iron phosphate 114
irritability 66, 67, 110, 111, 115, 120, 121, 124, 130
    in children 72, 94

J
jealousy 67
joints 85, 104, 126

K
Kent, Dr James Tyler 32
kidneys 66

L
Lachesis 58, 66, 67, *82* 91, **119**
lack of self-confidence 83
lack of stamina 130
lactose 96
larkspur 131
laryngitis 109, 131
Law of Similars 11, 12
Ledum (Ledum palustre) 88, 93, **120**
ligaments 93
liver problems 20, 122, 125
loneliness 67, 84, 102
low energy 120, 133
lower back pain 128
lung problems 78, 101
Lycopodium 58, 59, 62, 67, 75, 83, 89, 120
    constitutional type **38-9**

M
Magnesia phosphorica Mag phos) 72, **121**
magnesium 121
"maintaining causes" 21
malaria 11, 12, 110
mandrake 125
marigold 107
marsh tea 120
mastitis **68**, 124
Materia Medica 12, 50, 96
may apple 125
measles 27, **76**, 102, 104, 114
menopause **66**
menstrual problems 111, 126, 130
menthol 59
Mercurius 57, 58, 59, 71, 73, 77, 94, **121**
mercury 121
minerals 65
modalities 48-9
moisturizing creams 74
monkshood 100
mood swings 44, 66, 75, 116, 126, 127
morning sickness 119, 130
motor nerves 114
mouth ulcers 121
mucous membranes 101, 111, 128, 129
mucus (phlegm) 56, 59, 78, 101
mumps 27, 77, 102, 121, 126
muscular problems 83, 103, 114, 128

N
nasal discharge 59, 73, 81
Natrum muriaticum (Nat mur) 13, 67, 75, 81, 84, **122**
    constitutional type **40-***1*
Natrum sulphuricum (Nat sulph) 70, 80, **122**
nausea 62, **63**, 111, 113, 119, 124, 130
neck problems 56, 59, 63
nerve pain 87, 93, 116
nervousness 83, 102
nervous system 109, 110, 128
nightmares 75
nipples 68, 124
nosebleeds 42, **91**, 112, 124

nostrils, blocked 81
nutrients 24, 25, 124
Nux vomica 62, 63, **124**

O
oedema 102
oils 52, 73, 137
oral herpes 122
Organon, The 11
ovaries 77
oyster shells 32, 33, 106

P
panic attacks 83, 102
pasque flower 126
perennial rhinitis 81
period pains 67, 111, 121
peritonitis 62
pertussis *see* whooping cough
Peruvian bark 110
phobias 83
Phosphorus 57, 61, 63, 83, 91, 93, **124**
    constitutional type **42-3**
Phytolacca 58, 68, **125**
piles *see* haemorrhoids
pimples 135
Podophyllum 61, **125**
poison ivy 126
poison-nut tree 124
poisons 133
poke root 125
pollen 80, 81, 129
pollution 28
potassium bisulphate 109
potencies 14-15, 50, 51, 96
precautions, general 51
pregnancy 51, 74, 115, 119, 130
premenstrual tension (PMT) 67, 119
prescribing
    for children **32-47**
    at home 16-17, 20, 34, 139
prickly heat 136
prolapse 130
provings 12
psoriasis 74
Pulsatilla 57, 59, 61, 84, 89, 90, 94, 98,
126, *127*
    childhood 70, 71, 73, 74, 75, 76, 77
    constitutional type **44-5**
    respiratory 80, 81
    women's problems 66, 67, 68
puncture wounds 88, 120
pupils, dilated 58, 76
pus *see* discharges

Q
quicksilver 121
quinine 11-12, 110

R
rashes 76, 126
rectum 100

red onion 101
relaxation 22-3
remedies 17, 34, 51
    guide **96-139**
    index 50, 99
    wrong 17, 50
Rescue remedy 90, 92, **137**
respiratory system 36, 112, 119, 124, 131
restlessness 83, 121, 126
rhinitis 81
rhinovirus 55
Rhus tox (Rhus toxicodendron) 57, 71, *85*,
93, **126**
rubella **74**
rue **128**
Rumex **128**
Ruta 87, 88, 91, 93, 96, 97, **128**

S
Sabadilla 81, **129**
St Ignatius' bean 116
St John's wort 116
saliva increase 121
salt 13
Sarsaparilla 66, **129**
scalds 87, 107
sciatica 121
self-healing 14, 18, 22, 26-7, 28, 31, 54
sensitivity 83, 110, 130
Sepia 66, 67, **130**
sepsis 107, 115, 121
shingles 71, 126
shock 87, 90, **92**, 103, 116, 137
Silica 59, 94, **130**
silver nitrate 102
sinusitis 59
skin problems 15, 46, 88, 133, 135, 136
sodium chloride 122
sores **88**, 107
sore throat 58, 100, 102, 104, 106, 115,
119, 120, 121, 124, 131
Spanish fly 107
Spongia 56, 72, **131**
spots 135
sprains 85, **93**, 126, 128
Staphysagria 66, 84, 89, 92, 93, **131**
stinging nettle 136
stings *see* bites and stings
stomach pains 61, 62, 104, 111, 112, 120
stools, bloody 63
strains 85, **93**, 126
Streptococcus 58
stress 21-2, 89, 111, 131
stubbornness 106
styes 44, **89**, 131
succussion 14, 96
Sulphur 63, 89, *132*, **133**
    constitutional type **46-7**
sunburn **87**, 107
sundew 112
surgery effects **93**, 131
susceptibility 20

sweating 101, 110, 112, 115, 121
swollen glands 57, 73, 77, 106, 121, 126
swollen joints 85
Symphytum 8, 9, 91, 106, **133**
symptom patterns 8, 15, 35, 48, 73, 96
    in children **36, 38, 40, 42, 44, 46**

T
Tabacum 95, **135**
tantrums 75
tarantula spider *134*, 135
Tarentula cubensis (Tarent cub) *134*, **135**
teething problems 75, 77, 110, 126
temperature, body 56, 58, 77
tendons 93, 128
testicles 77
thoroughwort 113
tiredness 90, 114
tobacco plant 135
tonsillitis 58, 115, 119, 121, 124
toothache **94**, 104, 115, 121, 130
tooth extraction 93
totality of symptoms 16
toxins 27, 30, 61, 133
trauma 92, 93, 116
travel sickness **95**, 111, 135
treatments **48-95**

U
ulcers 110
unconsciousness 90
urethra 107
urinary system 66, 107, 129
Urtica 87, **136**
urticaria 136

V
veins, engorged 100, 115
Veratrum album 61, 63, **136**
Verbascum 52, 73, **137**
viral illnesses 55, 77
vision problems 88
vital force 15, 16, 31
vomiting **63**, 110, 111, 112, 119, 124, 136

W
weepiness 66, 67, 84, 126
white bryony 104
whooping cough 78, 111, 112, 119
wild rosemary 120
wild yam 113
witch hazel 115
women's problems 53, **65-8**
worry 102, 103, 114
wounds 107, 110, 130, 131
wrong remedies 17, 50

Y
yellow dock 128
yellow jasmine 114